CONVICTION

Conviction

The Making and Unmaking of the Violent Brain

OLIVER ROLLINS

STANFORD UNIVERSITY PRESS
Stanford, California

STANFORD UNIVERSITY PRESS
Stanford, California

Printed in the United States of America on acid-free, archival-quality paper

Library of Congress Cataloging-in-Publication Data
Names: Rollins, Oliver, author.
Title: Conviction : the making and unmaking of the violent brain /
    Oliver Rollins.
Description: Stanford, California : Stanford University Press, 2021. |
    Includes bibliographical references and index.
Identifiers: LCCN 2020044693 (print) | LCCN 2020044694 (ebook) |
    ISBN 9781503607019 (cloth) | ISBN 9781503627895 (paperback) |
    ISBN 9781503627901 (ebook)
Subjects: LCSH: Violence—Physiological aspects. | Neurosciences—
    Moral and ethical aspects. | Neurosciences—Social aspects.
Classification: LCC RC569.5.V55 R65 2021 (print) | LCC RC569.5.V55 (ebook) |
    DDC 612.8—dc23
LC record available at https://lccn.loc.gov/2020044693
LC ebook record available at https://lccn.loc.gov/2020044694

Cover design: Rob Ehle

Cover photo: iStockphoto | yngsa (@boyskyi)

Text design: Kevin Barrett Kane

Typeset at Stanford University Press in 10/14.4 Minion Pro

Contents

Preface

Of the Meaning of (Scientific) Progress

When I was growing up, I always wanted to be a physician. That was my dream, my own little symbol of progress. We need more black doctors, I would say, as I tried to assure myself that majoring in biology was the best choice. As I was just finishing my bachelor's degree, however, I realized that the biological sciences did not satisfy my thirst for knowledge in areas that were increasingly affecting my life. Luckily, I had been introduced to Africana (Black) Studies during undergrad as well, which opened my eyes to questions about health and race in a much different light. Racism and inequality are not just visible barriers to healthy living; they are "fundamental causes" of disparities, systemic social mechanisms that operate in a routinized fashion.[1] After completing my bachelor's, I left the biological sciences to pursue a master's in Pan-African Studies. It was during this time that the shape of what would become this book project started to emerge.

In the course of my research, I came across a staggering statistic: homicide was the leading cause of death for African American men ages 15–34.[2] That figure still holds true today. Pause and think about that for a minute. To place it in perspective: this subgroup of African American men is the *only* part of the U.S. population for whom this holds true. Homicide accounts for 50 percent of deaths among young African American men ages 15–19 each year, yet we overwhelmingly turn to the criminal justice system for answers to this "problem." But why? How can this dramatic loss of young lives be a problem primarily for the police or the courts to handle? At that time, as a 25-year-old black male born and raised in the U.S. South, I quickly realized that I needed to adjust my own perspective and regard the situation as a "health problem," refocusing my attention on the well-being of young people who are readily overlooked in society.

I hoped that if I reframed violence as a health problem, my research would be useful for developing more-effective violence-prevention strategies for racially marginalized communities. Instead of understanding violence as a problem with penological solutions that emphasize incarceration and punishment as deterrents, regarding it as a health problem stresses the need to build safer, healthier people and communities by addressing the deep social inequities that disproportionately affect racially marginalized populations. To be clear, my transition to viewing violence as a health problem should not be confused with a search for innate causes of it within the body. However, the ongoing research into the issue increasingly emphasized the need to identify and examine defective genes and abnormal brains for new clues about violence. The focus on genetics and neuroscience took me back to a familiar place—the biological sciences—and ultimately what had begun as an exploration of violence prevention turned into a study of the construction and politics of scientific knowledge—examining the formative role that race plays in the making of health research, and the societal consequences.

While developing this project, I was aware of the well-established body of social science literature on the "molecularization of race" in the post-genomic age.[3] We know now that the completion of the Human Genome Project in 2001 did not signal the end of race as a scientific question. Genetic research, we learned, regularly treated race as a fixed biological fact instead of as the contingent, fluid, sociopolitical concept that it is.[4] New scientific questions on health, behavior, and identity often reflect well-worn biologized ideas of racial difference.[5] Thus, neither the ubiquity of race as an "old" scientific question nor the continued debate over its use or meaning in "new" biological research has occurred by accident.

This book developed from a similar curiosity about the treatment of race in contemporary neuroscientific research. I wanted to understand how neuroscientists use race (and ethnicity), how they interpret racial (and ethnic) differences in results and navigate the potential racial impacts of these knowledges once they travel out of the lab. Did neuroscientists struggle, like their genetic counterparts, to address the ongoing challenges of the (neuro) biologization of race? Given that neuropsychologists were already responding to skeptics, both within and outside the field, who viewed the growing use of neuroimaging as "modern phrenology," how were they dealing with other related (and troublesome) legacies of the science, like scientific racism?[6] Did neuroimaging, with its technological promise to "see" the biological underpinnings of social life, warrant special ethical attention when considering differences in brain structure or neural circuitry between racial or ethnic social groupings?

In an attempt to take up sociologist Troy Duster's challenge to investigate the intricate relationships between science and race at the site of knowledge production, my ideal venue for exploring these questions was the neuroscience of violence.[7] As I thought at the time, "How can neuroscientists truly comprehend the underpinnings of violence without considering how the *effects of race* influence the discernment of and response to such behaviors in society?" Historically, biological research on violent behaviors had been especially fraught with social, ethical, and political dilemmas concerning race and racism. Violence and racism are intricately connected social facts. This is especially true in U.S. society, where historical and ongoing systemic practices of race, ethnicity, and inequality are complexly entangled with sociocultural perceptions of dangerousness, citizenship, and criminality, alongside sociopolitical enactments of policing, stigmatization, and surveillance.[8] Furthermore, the new biology of violence seems also to frame violence as a health problem. How are brain scans capturing environmental and structural consequences of racism, I wondered? And, importantly, can a science, and scientific technologies, engage with such dynamics if it mainly seeks to uncover molecular processes taking place under the skull?

In the end, however, this book did not turn out to be focused solely on neuroscience and race—although this is not to imply that race is inconsequential to brain studies on violence. Early in the project I discovered that race was playing a discursively haunting role on this science, which complicated my efforts to uncover its use and impact. First, contrary to my original thinking, the neuroscience of violence does *not* talk about race in any blatant manner. The term "race" (or "ethnicity") is usually relegated to truncated mentions, if any, about research participants in demographic tables of articles. Even more rare are discussions about racism, which appear in a handful of books by researchers, but mostly in reference to the program's past. It was a relief to know that today's neuroscientists were not encouraging the same racist claims of past biocriminology. However, this finding deepened my concerns about the potential ways race could affect this science. If researchers are not willing to write about race or racism, how can we be sure that they have addressed such issues?

Second, it was becoming clear that securing interviews with neuroscientists who researched violence would be a challenge. I am a qualitative sociologist, so I was fully aware of the potential logistical difficulties and frustrations that come with interviewing. I used multiple methods to collect data for this project: analysis of published research; participant observation; academic coursework in neuroscience; and interviews with neuropsychologists who were studying violence. Many of my questions could be addressed with the first three sources, but interviews were becoming more vital, given that, as mentioned above, this field of research rarely discusses race in publications.

To be clear, I do not think that the hesitancy to participate by some neuroscientists was simply a question of my race, and the neuroscientists I spoke to quickly denounced antiquated racist understandings of biology and violence. However, being a black man asking questions about race and violence certainly did not make it easier to secure interviews. In fact, one interviewee later informed me that many other neuroscientists would turn down my requests to participate because discussions about race, or even the ethics of such research, were too politically volatile.[9] It is fair to believe that these neuroscientists, particularly those based in the United States, might have viewed my project as too risky, fearing that their replies or research might be misperceived as racially insensitive. However, what does it mean for these neuroscientists to retreat from discussions about the social and ethical repercussions of race and racism, when these issues undergird a significant portion of the scrutiny toward such research in the first place? Thus, the new biology of violence is different from that which came before, but so far it has been unsuccessful in exorcising the ghosts of its racist past.

Thinking more deeply about how to capture the work of race on/in this science, I pivoted to a different but tangential subject: the "question of progress." We are told that science is objective, rational, and transformative, and this is why the production of scientific knowledge will inevitably improve our lives. If science is progressing, just where is it going? Who gets to shape this narrative? And to what end? Moreover, was this strategy toward race supposed to be an example of scientific progress—a science that seeks to operate in a racially "color-blind" fashion?[10]

Society needs scientific progress, we are advised. Each new scientific advancement supposedly corresponds to observable improvements in health, behavior, technology, and social life; thus, science *is* progress. Scholars in science and technology studies have long been critical of narratives that convey a natural progression of scientific inquiry.[11] Rejecting the idea that scientific progress is a linear, objective, and/or natural process, these scholars make clear that the production of scientific knowledge is a human or social practice, and that scientific progress is neither a straightforward accumulation of knowledge nor an obvious development of thought.

Yet, my reference point for progress began elsewhere, in the sociology of race with contributions from scholars like W.E.B. Du Bois, who reminded us of "the sobering realization of the meaning [and limits] of progress."[12] Sociologists examining the significance and function of the "question of race" have critically assessed the optimal properties, continued struggles, and failures of social progress. Such scholarship pushes back against barriers to justice and equality. Moreover, these accounts operate as a space of resistance, an arena in which to imagine counternarratives to the normative accounts of progress that often exclude the voices of the marginalized, vulnerable, and oppressed. Through these analyses we better understand that there is nothing inevitable, nor inherently liberating, about social progress in our society. "Progress is necessarily ugly," Du Bois would write.[13]

Slightly shifting my focus, and retooling my analytic lens, I began to think about the way narratives of scientific progress resonate with, and are *coproduced* through, existing visions of social progress.[14] This is evident when considering attempts by scientists to create, often uncritically, "race-neutral" research—ostensibly an indication of bioethical growth and awareness—which mirror many of the sociocultural and political responses toward race and racism at the end of the twentieth century. Therefore, though this book may not be directly about race, the acumen and dexterity of racial theory—helping me make sense of how racial *difference* actually works in society, how racial *inequality* remains salient, and how the *power* of race can "manufacture futures"—created the space I needed to write it.[15]

Placing these narratives in conversation, reflexively, helped me better realize the inextricable relationship between controversy and progress. And so it became clear that progress is an antiquated, crude, and normalizing paradigm. Adherence to this kind of perfunctory reading of progress leaves us woefully unprepared to capture either the incessant function of racial relations or the politics of scientific knowledges and technologies. Furthermore, I'm suggesting that the normative ideas that underpin what we call progress, social and scientific, thought to axiomatically bend "the arc of the moral universe" toward justice and freedom, or reason and truth, can help reconstitute power dynamics. My goal, therefore, is not to prove or disprove the scientific validity of the neuroscience of violence. Questions about whether such research is real science or pseudoscience present a false dichotomy that dehistoricizes and decontextualizes the social contingencies that go into the making of all scientific innovation and obscure the actual biopolitical domains that help organize the production of knowledge. Instead, *Conviction* offers a fresh understanding regarding the endurance and seeming necessity of biological understandings for behavior, as well as the persistent and often convincing backlash against such knowledges of violence.

This branch of science has never demonstrated how its pursuit of progress—use of advanced scientific technologies, revised ontological purchase, and new ethical observances—constitutes a more socially useful way to "know" violence. Duster urges us to pay close attention to the way certain ontologies about violent subjects remain central to this research program.[16] Here, I aim to show that certain normative assumptions about difference, inequality, and power that operate in a systemic fashion in society are actually embedded, unrecognized by researchers, in the making, practice, and promises of the neuroscience of violence. I therefore contend that this new neurobiological model of "violence as a health problem" remains problematic, as it inadequately comprehends the role of social inequality, and therefore undermines researchers' stated goal of producing a complete "picture" of and effective intervention for violence.

Acknowledgments

This is my first book. Book writing is no easy task. It can be a strenuous and often isolated journey toward completion. Still, my journey, like so many others, was filled with, and only made possible through, an enormous amount of support. I want to start by thanking Howard Pinderhughes, who continues to be instrumental to my growth as scholar. Howard models what it takes to be both a scholar and social activist, and I am so gracious for his unwavering support and advice. He was the first person to tell me I was asking a compelling question, and his early guidance stuck with me throughout in this process. Without a doubt, this book would have not been complete without his support. Similarly, I continue to be in awe of the brilliance of Janet Shim. Janet sharpened my thinking as a grad student while at the University of California, San Francisco. Her impeccable instruction taught me how to seriously engage social theory, and sociology as a whole. Thus, I owe so much of my intellectual development to her stellar mentorship and teaching, and I cannot imagine getting to this point in my life with her extraordinary insights and encouragement. Adele Clarke introduced me to science, technology, and medicine studies (STMS), and without question she was invaluable to this project. I cannot thank Adele enough for her meetings and discussions about this project, and her support of me even when I could not envision fully what this project was supposed to be or do. Moreover,

I'm especially grateful for her extremely astute, purple inked, marked-up versions of my early drafts of this manuscript (If you have ever received Adele's magnificent hand-written editorial comments, you know what I'm talking about!) Troy Duster's scholarship laid the foundation for this book. Anyone who knows Troy knows that he has a way of challenging you, and compelling you do your best work, through a straightforward, yet immensely compelling and exhilarating, dialogue. His advice to me from the beginning was to not to let the novelty of the brain sciences overshadow the way old logics of difference and inequality continue to find ways to operate through contemporary knowledges and technologies. Without a doubt, I kept this in mind through my writing of the book, and I hope my presentation of the "Dusterian" perspective meets Troy's expectations. I also owe much gratitude to Osagie Obasogie for listening to and reading through early formulations of this project. Osagie's expertise in law, bioscience, and ethics shaped my take on the potential ethical impacts of neuroscientific interventions for violence, and it encouraged me to deepen my understanding of the complexly entangle relationship between law and neuroscience.

Conviction came together during my postdoc in Penn's Program on Race, Science & Society (PRSS). Under the leadership of Dorothy Roberts, PRSS is devoted to promoting interdisciplinary understanding of, and dispelling myths about, the role of race in scientific research. Dorothy Roberts's mentoring has been nothing less than amazing. Dorothy has a way of guiding and supporting you well before you come to recognize it, and she always went over and beyond to ensure everything I needed to succeed. Through her support, PRSS provided the space I needed for my ideas to mature. Her dedication to social justice, which she also instills in each of her mentees, inspired me to restructure the final form of this manuscript and focus distinctly on the normative impacts of social inequality. As a PRSS postdoc, I was also fortunate to be surround by an outstanding cohort of post-doc colleagues in Penn's Center for Africana Studies. Seriously, Grace Sanders-Johnson, Alden Young, Clemmie Harris, Amber Reed, and Dhanveer Brar, you are all amazing. In just a short time, we worked diligently as a team to craft our book proposals, give each other feedback and advice, and be there in support for each other no matter the issue. In the end, all of us received book contracts. Moreover, I'm so grateful for the exceptionally welcoming scholarly environment from Penn's Center for Africana Studies, including staff Carol Davis, Teya Campbell, and Gale Garrison, and the support and wisdom from Camille Charles, Michael Hanchard, Deborah Thomas, Barbara Savage, Eve Trout Powell, Tukufu Zuberi and Heather Williams. I am truly indebted to Heather, whose office door was always open when I needed advice, and for her comments on an early draft of the book proposal. Moreover, my periodic lunch meetings with Tukufu were instrumental in formulating my theoretical and empirical understanding of the operation and meaning of race as a social process, which are not only key to this book, but also my current projects on race and neuroscience.

This book could not have been writing without the participants in the study. I would like to thank all the neuroscientists that sat down for interviews, and graciously shared their expertise about the neuroscience of violence and antisocial behavior. Also, thanks to Martha Farah, who served as my mentor during my time in Penn's Center for Neuroscience and Society, Geoffrey Aguirre, and Penn's Neuroscience Boot Camp; all essential in advancing my understanding of neuroimaging technologies and neuroethics. Moreover, I am very appreciative of my informal conversations at Penn with Adrian Raine, who was kind enough to share his views about the historical and contemporary issues surrounding the neuroscience of violence, and for inviting me to share my early thoughts on this project with his graduate class.

Early versions of chapters from *Conviction* were presented to several different audiences. I would like to thank UC Berkeley's Center for Race and Gender; Penn's Department of Africana Studies, History and Sociology of Science, and Center for Neuroscience and Society; Drexel's Public Health and Science and Technology Program; University of Houston's African American Studies Program; Wesleyan University's Science in Society Program, Princeton's Department of African American Studies, and the University of Louisville's Discourse and Semiotics Workshop. Similarly, I want to acknowledge the support and guidance I received from California Science and Technology Studies (STS) Retreat, Kathy Charmaz's Qualitative Research Writing Workshop at UCSF, and *Symbioses: Biosocial Research Network Group*. Notably, I am beyond fortunate for the funding support for this project from National Institute of General Medical Sciences (NIGMS), Initiative for Maximizing Student Diversity (IMSD) Fellowship (1-R25-GM56847); National Institutes of Health (NIH), National Human Genome Research Institute (NHGRI), The Ethical, Legal, and Social Implications (ELSI) Research Program, Supplement to Promote Diversity Health Related Research (RO1-HG115848–03S1); UCSF Graduate Division, Rosenberg-Hill Graduate Research Fellowship; University of California, Center for New Racial Studies (UCCNRS) Graduate Research Grant; Penn's Program on Race, Science & Society and Center for Africana Studies; and the University of Louisville's College of Arts and Science.

So much of this book took shape through conversations, and there are several colleagues that I would like to thank for pushing me to refine my ideas in science and technology studies (STS). Conversations with Aaron Panofsky, Ruha Benjamin, Alondra Nelson, Anthony Hatch, Victoria Pitts-Taylor, Jenny Reardon, Kate Darling, Krista Sigurdson, Sonia Rab Alam, Christopher Hanssmann, Martine Lappé, Taylor Cruz, Joe Dumit, Susan Lindee, Anna Jabloner, Kelly Joyce, Michael Yudell, Susan Bell, Chole Silverman, Katrina Karkazis, Projit Mukherji, and Debjani Bhattacharyya helped shape the various viewpoints that made it into the book. I am particularly appreciative of the detailed exchanges, scholarly suggestions, and ongoing co-authorship, about race, crime, and biomedical technologies with Torsten Voigt, Julien Larregue, and Lee Young. In addition, I cherish my illuminating talks throughout this process with Jamie Chang, Jennifer Nazareno, Jarmin Yeh, Dani Holtz, Craig Franson, Raha Rafii, Kevin Jenkins, Ben Wiggins, Natalie Ingraham, David Peterson, Latonia Craig, Floyd Craig, Stacy Brooks, Lucie Brooks, Elizabeth Jones, Deonte Hollowell, Amari Johnson, and Tabea Cornel. Likewise, my writing group at the University of Louisville, Melanie Gast, Cynthia Ganote, Anna Ribeiro Browne, Frank Kelderman, Angela Storey, and Andrea Olinger, provided another collegial and supported space that helped me push this book across the finish line. Moreover, thanks to my other colleagues at the University of Louisville who welcomed me to campus, and helped navigate my first few years as an assistant professor, during the writing of this book, especially Latrica Best, Carson Byrd, Theresa Rajack-Tally, Ricky Jones, Karen Christopher, Michal Kofman, Lauren Heberle, Michelle Foster, Gul Marshall, Dave Roelfs, Avery Kolers, Lisa Bjorkman, and James Conyers (University of Houston). Furthermore, I owe much to Martyn Pickersgill. It goes without saying that Martyn's scholarship on the sociology of neuroscience was imperative for this book. However, I'm also much obliged for his thoughtful advice during the early stages of this project, and particularly his willingness to provide detailed comments and suggestions on an early version of the entire book manuscript! Martyn's advices helped me identify the tension and short-comings in the early draft, which I drew upon extensively to help restructure the final organization and presentation of the book. And, a very special thanks to Catherine Bliss. Rina generously introduced me to the editors at Stanford University Press, and answered all the questions I had to help me begin and navigate the publication process. Thus, Rina paved the path for the product you read today!

I am honored to have my book published with Stanford University Press (SUP), and I want thank my outstanding editor Marcela Maxfield for her insightful comments, suggestions, and encouragement throughout this jour-ney. I would also like to thank SUP Editor-in-Chief Kate Wahl, who took the time to personally work with and comment on the early versions of the book proposal. She believed in the project from the start, and I owe her much for her early trust in me and faith in this book project. Thanks also goes to the excellent SUP production team, particularly Emily Smith, and especially her patience in the final stages of the book process, and my amazing copy-editor Jan McInroy.

Finally, I must thank my family. My mother who has always provided support and motivation I have needed to push through the most challeng-ing obstacles in my life. Moreover, I am forever beholden to my dad, sister, brother, nieces, nephew, cousins, aunts, uncles, and friends. Neither this book, nor my path in academia, were possible without their extraordinary and steadfast encouragement and love. The pleasure I felt at the completion of this book project was an extension of the joy, happiness, and inspiration I received from them throughout this long journey.

CONVICTION

PART I

THE MAKING OF THE VIOLENT BRAIN

1 | BIOLOGY, VIOLENCE, AND THE CONTINUED DEBATE

IN APRIL 1997, *U.S. News & World Report* released an issue of its long-running weekly magazine featuring an article titled "Politics of Biology." Written by scientific journalist Wray Herbert, "Politics of Biology" is a brief yet well-informed commentary on the stakes surrounding what Herbert called the "biologization of American culture."[1] Yet, even before turning to read Herbert's essay, audiences were immediately struck, if not disturbed, by the magazine's cover image of a toddler dressed in a miniature black-and-white prison-striped jumpsuit with a matching cap. Printed across the child's torso, in a bold white font, was a single question: "Born Bad?"[2] The provocative image and the rhetorical query that accompanied it were seemingly intended to tug at the audience's sensibilities, indirectly encouraging them to grapple with the deeper societal purpose and consequences of being "born bad." As noted in the closing words of Herbert's article,

> So, assume for a minute that there is a cluster of genes somehow associated with youthful violence. The kid who carries those genes might inhabit a world of loving parents, regular nutritious meals, lots of books, safe schools. Or his [*sic*] world might be a world of peeling paint and gunshots around the corner. In which environment would those genes be likely to manufacture the biochemical underpinnings of criminality? Or for that matter, the proteins and synapses of happiness?[3]

Further questioning is required to accurately capture the salience of Herbert's statements. What are these supposed genetic links among biological inheritance and criminal behaviors? And how does one's "environment" factor into this biological explanation? Critically, how will scientists detect, and accurately *know*, who is born bad? For that matter, what are we, as a society, being asked to do if they "discover" biological proof that the cute toddler in the prison-striped onesie may be destined for a life of crime?

While it is difficult to pin down an exact date for the emergence of this mode of inquiry, scholars often point to Italian physician Cesare Lombroso's "criminal anthropology" in the late nineteenth century as a pivotal point for the evolution of the biology of violence.[4] Research on biology and violence never regained the popularity it had during Lombroso's heyday; nevertheless, a steadily increasing body of research seeking to find the true underpinnings of the "born criminal" thesis continues to this day. At the same time, critics from the academic, biomedical, legal, and public spheres have argued that attempts to uncover the biological roots of violence threaten philosophical doctrines like free will and personal responsibility, erroneously label crime a medical illness, stigmatize individuals deemed violent or psychologically impaired, and reinforce racist and eugenic discourses that help to justify existing inequalities in society.[5] Starting in the late 1980s, however, a different approach to biology and violence was proposed, one that sought to eschew the technical, social, and ethical flaws that had plagued past versions of this research.

The latest efforts to uncover biological determinants of violence reflect the scientific breakthroughs that gave rise to modern-day genetics and the neurosciences. In general, the rise of neuroscience and genetic technologies helped to shift biomedical understandings of the human body away from blood, organs, and hormones to identification and manipulation of health through molecular-level mechanisms and biochemical functions.[6] Genetic- and brain-based investigations of crime existed well before the late 1980s. However, the molecular era restored a sense of "technological optimism" for contemporary researchers in the biology of violence,[7] who hoped that molecular-era science could finally deliver the definitive proof of the biological underpinnings of behavior that eluded the likes of Lombroso and others. The adoption of these new technologies, however, did little to quell critics' suspicions that the "new" biocriminology was just "old wine in new bottles."[8]

A considerable portion of this criticism was aimed at genetic research on violence, which was somewhat expected, given the pervasiveness of "gene talk" during the 1990s.[9] Popular images and media narratives helped to translate the molecular language of genetics into everyday discussions, which convincingly conveyed the presumed powers of the gene. According to sociologist Dorothy Nelkin and historian Susan Lindee, this new and pervasive cultural message of "genetic essentialism . . . equate[d] human beings, in their social, historical, and moral complexity, with their genes."[10] As researchers began to utilize molecular genetics to study crime, critics issued their own counter-messages that warned of the latent dangers of biologization. Moreover, they had reason for concern.

Five years before the "born bad" article, alarms were raised about a proposed, and subsequently canceled, U.S. National Institutes of Health (NIH)-sponsored conference on the genetics of crime. Opponents framed the would-be conference as a veiled endorsement of racist ideas about the nature of violence. These accusations were leveraged by the ill-informed statements of Frederick Goodwin, then director of the Alcohol, Drug Abuse, and Mental Health Administration. In a speech earlier that year, Goodwin referred to inner-city urban areas as "jungles" and suggested that violence committed by African American youths was synonymous with behavior of the so-called hyper-aggressive, hyper-sexualized rhesus monkey.[11] Shortly after the conference fiasco, the publication of *The Bell Curve* in 1995 further stirred up the clouds of racial controversy surrounding genetic research, due to its authors' claims that intelligence was both genetic and variable by race, which critics quickly lambasted as another case of genetic determinism and scientific racism.[12] Moreover, such concerns persisted into the following decade, as the completion of the Human Genome Project (HGP) helped expand research on genetics and violence, and penal systems increased their dependency on DNA forensic technologies.[13] Strikingly, though, very few of these critiques addressed the potential challenges of the *neuroscience of violence*, even though neuroimaging research on violent behaviors developed during the same time period as contemporary genetic research on violence did.

President George H. W. Bush actually designated the 1990s as the "Decade of the Brain." Following Congress's joint resolution of the same title, Bush's proclamation called for increased funding to "enhance public awareness of the benefits to be derived from brain research"—an objective shared by his

Democratic counterpart Barack Obama nearly twenty-three years later, who was optimistic that his own *BRAIN Initiative* would finally "unlock the mystery of the three pounds of matter that sits between our ears."[14] Throughout much of the decade, however, the fervor surrounding the HGP, and the promise of the gene, often overshadowed the Bush administration's aspirations for the brain. Still, the Decade of the Brain was transformative in its own right.

Neuroscience activities intensified the development and use of brain technologies in the hope of providing greater knowledge of and treatments for neurological diseases. Public awareness of brain research also improved, along with new policy agendas that supported increasing public funding for early childhood development.[15] Furthermore, one of the most important legacies of the Decade of the Brain was the enthusiasm for brain plasticity. The idea that the brain is a highly malleable composite of neuronal circuitry was not new; however, the notion took on a slightly different significance during the 1990s. Brains were not just changing but being shaped through our sociocultural experiences in the world.[16] The possibilities for brain research were suddenly even more appealing, and with it, a wider appreciation of a "we are our brains" ontology within the psychological (psy-) sciences.[17] Seemingly tucked away in this discursive shift to "brainhood," however, was the emergence of a new brain-based biology of violence.

Researchers in the neuroscience of violence constitute a relatively small group of neuroscientists. Like most neuroscientists today, the majority of these researchers were trained in the psy-sciences. My use of the term "neuroscientist" or "neuropsychologist," therefore, applies to researchers from any field who primarily employ neuroscientific techniques and technologies to explore the relationship between the brain and violence.[18] Neuroscientists studying violence have benefited from a significant increase in funding opportunities for neuro-related research on psychiatric disorders, which subsequently resulted in a steady rise in research on neurobiology and violence over the last thirty years. A few of the well-known neuroscientists in the field have built impressive public personas that have helped them to productively disseminate their work through media outlets and engage with public audiences. Moreover, some of the core research arguments produced here extend beyond the study of violence to address seemingly less-controversial or more-legitimate social questions and problems like altruism, childhood development, or maltreatment.[19]

Similar to other scientific fields, neuroscience carries no predetermined consensus of ideas. Thus there are important intradisciplinary disputes about the production, meaning, and use of neurobiological knowledges of violence. Not all researchers under the banner of neuroscience agree about what kinds of brain knowledges count as pertinent, what a neurobiological influence should or will look like, or even where and how to employ brain-based solutions for violence. Nevertheless, these collective differences are all bound by virtue of a recognition that neurobiological mechanisms allow for a more meticulous and complete interpretation of violence, and therefore constitute a new(er), yet still controversial, *research program*.

This research program, or simply "the program," refers to multiple academic disciplines, researchers, methodologies, and theories of violence or criminality, all of which are ontologically aligned through a specific set of principles—a "hard core"—about the causation of criminal or violent behavior.[20] Philosopher Ian Hacking characterizes the entire field of criminology as a *degeneracy research program*.[21] In his view, the degeneracy research program hinges on two central ideas about the origins of criminal behavior: an overall recognition that deviant types are profoundly antisocial due to "innate defect[s] in individuals" and that individuals inherit such deficiencies from a previous generation.[22] Although I agree with much of Hacking's characterization, in this book the term "research program" is limited to biological theories of violence.[23]

There is something new about this manifestation of the (neuro)biology of violence that differs from its criminological lineage and extends beyond the interpretive flexibility allowed for by the program's "protective belt."[24] The "new research program," as sociologist Nikolas Rose argues, is based on the "search for links between specific biological abnormalities and the propensity to commit violent crime, with a view to early identification, preventive intervention, and effective treatment."[25] The emphasis on "propensity," or *risk*, is key for the revival of the program in the mid-twentieth century, as this framework carved out a more pronounced ontological and epistemological space between the biology of violence and its criminology origins. While certain terminology and, to an extent, goals remain shared between criminology and the biology of violence, there are also important conceptual distinctions among criminologists, who are interested in biological variants to help complete existing theories of criminality, on the one hand, and neuropsychologists, who study the neurobiological and genetic mechanisms underlying mental disorder, on the other. This book's focus is on the latter, through which "a new molecular biopolitics of control is taking shape."[26]

Conviction has special meaning in this book. Readers might assume that neuroscientific data seek to identify criminals, and subsequently provide biological proof of their guilt. However, neuroscientists are less interested in detecting who is a criminal, or determining fault, innocence, or guilt. Moreover, they do not aim for neuro-knowledges to excuse criminally violent behaviors. The neurobiological argument, on its surface, seems to be a rather simple one: "Until we know as much about this inner dimension as we do about the outer one—what goes on inside the heads of aggressors and their victims—we are not prepared to analyze the problem of violence effectively."[27] Consequently, neurologists trust that their brain-based knowledges will provide crucial information about violence that would otherwise be unknown or unattainable. This approach has led to the creation of the *violent brain* model—a unique brain type thought to capture new kinds of violent subjects, *potential* criminals. It is their faith in this brain type that allows this book to view conviction as a means to illuminate neuroscientific motivation, trust, and defense of neurobiological logics of violence. And, therefore, this book pays close attention to the way "conviction functions as [an] ideological condition of possibility" for the construct I call the violent brain.[28]

Reviewing the emergence of neuroethics, historian Fernando Vidal argues that the subdiscipline's claim of autonomy and specificity from the traditional field of bioethics was established and maintained through its practitioners' deeply held belief that the neurosciences are exceptional, in the sense that their unparalleled access to the mind through its neurobiological underpinnings necessitates a unique class of ethics. For Vidal, conviction captures how neuroethics justifies its purpose in, and relationship to, the brain sciences and society, through the belief that the neurosciences will dramatically illuminate and improve upon human life in ways never seen before. In Vidal's words, neuroethics "has been justified by the *conviction*, sustained since the 1990s by the capability attributed to neuroimaging technologies, that somehow 'the mind is the brain.'"[29] In a related manner, I observe how conviction creates, facilitates, and expends belief in this construct, the violent brain, and in turn how neuroscientists operationalize these new knowledges to help manage the uncertainty, complexity, and controversy that the program continues to face. The use of the term "conviction" here captures the ontological commitment to the doctrine that the "mind is the brain," as well as the ongoing and coproduced nature of the research—that is, the tension between demonstrating scientific authority and exceptionalism on the one hand, and social and ethical purpose and potential on the other.[30]

Conviction traces the emergence of the neuroscience of violence and shows how neuroscientists navigate ongoing social and ethical concerns about the research program. This examination is based on an extensive qualitative content analysis of more than 300 peer-reviewed research articles and reviews on neuroimaging research on violence (circa 1990–2018). These data were further informed by interviews with 15 neuroscientists who focus on the study of violence. I also employed participant observation at neuroscience conferences/ workshops and enrolled in academic coursework and training covering such topics as social neuroscience, neuroethics, and neuroimaging research design and statistics. Collectively, this structured multimodal methodology illuminated the way the science is produced, contested, and rationalized. The "conditions of possibilities" surrounding the making of the neuroscience of violence paint an interesting sociological picture. The adoption of advanced scientific technologies and the remaking of the program's theoretical warrant operate as intricate sites of (re)production and legitimation that help make, explain, and substantiate the (continued) need, at least in the eyes of the producers of this knowledge, for neuroscientific research on violence. However, such contemporary shifts in the research program also affect the types of "cerebral subjects" that neuroscientists are expected to discover, the kinds of behaviors identified and fixed for inspection, and, as we will see, surveillance, via neuroscientific explanation. This, of course, requires further inquiry, to understand the threat or potential that these new neurobiological knowledges of violence pose for society. That is, why should we pay attention to, and be cautious of, this relatively select area of neuroscience in the first place? Below, I attempt to answer this question by focusing on the way the newest rendition of the biology of violence has embraced the "social" as an imperative element of neuroscientific knowledge and analysis. My interest, however, is not to debate whether neuroscientists truly believe that violence is a social, partly social, or biosocial behavior. Instead, I want to illuminate the work of the "social" or "biosocial" episteme in the ongoing debate about biology and violence. Specifically, how does this (messy) reading of the social brain take shape and become further refined and remade into a seemingly universal and bioethical response to controversy, and an ostensibly apolitical means to demonstrate and justify the social value and worth of brain knowledges of violence in society?

CONTROVERSY (STILL) MATTERS

Controversy has a central role in this story. Given the turbulent past and egregiously questionable applications of this "failed science," why have neuroscientists continued to pursue it?[31] Criticism of the biology of violence has been consistent. And while it seems as if the program has simply ignored these warnings about determinism, sexism, racism, and social control, a closer look at the program's persistence reveals a constant engagement with such debates. The research program, therefore, has endured and even thrived because of, and not despite, its notorious legacy.

In his examination of the development of behavioral genetics, sociologist Aaron Panofsky notes, "Controversy is persistent and ungovernable. . . . [It can] wax and wane or emerge explosively, but never really resolve and always threaten[s] to reappear."[32] Panofsky's words also apply to neurobiological perspectives of violence. Ordinarily, we might expect that continued controversy harms the research today—and it has, to an extent. However, controversy has more often been productive, if not vital, to the biology of violence. It operates as a dimension of the science, actively and continually shaping the production, appearance, and anticipated impression of research in this domain. In this way, neuroscientists are "using the past to help demarcate a contemporary regime of truth, to police the present, and to try to shape the future."[33] Neuroscientists are actively in conversation with their critics, even if unarticulated, and therefore, today's brain-based perspectives on violence are not new ideas that have been objectively discovered nor are they detected from sociocultural or historical meanings. Instead, the violent brain model has been designed, remade, and reshaped with the program's historical criticisms in mind. Let us place the program under a different analysis, one that emphasizes the work done through the invocation of the program's historical criticisms and rebuttals to expand this argument.[34]

There is an implicit heuristic function in the way neuroscientists often talk about and draw attention to particular kinds of errors of biocriminology. "A new generation of scientists are coming up who are much more focused and careful about how they assess things, how they define things, and how they quantify things. There's been truly a shift in our understanding of [violence]," neuropsychologist Dr. Lewis told me in our interview.[35] The idea that today's science better assesses violence suggests that the controversy about earlier biocriminology was simply due to empirical problems that are seemingly implausible today because of technological and ethical progress. However, if we consider the heuristic value of this statement, we can ascertain a different reading about the past. Neuroscientists indirectly leverage—rework, reproduce, and extend—certain ideas from the past through the research practices of today. To demonstrate, let's turn to the way certain ontological properties of the old program are retained in these new measures of violence.

The biology of violence has operated, and continues to operate, on the idea that new biological observations, measurements, or substrates will enable researchers to neatly separate the "violent" from the "normal" into two clear categories.[36] Historically, the program made these distinctions through "pseudoscientific" measurements of outer bodily traits, and today we see these differences upheld at the molecular level in more-legitimate scientific practices to help render the science empirical and doable. In theory, the neuroscience of violence considers the violent (criminal or antisocial) and the normal as two distinct kinds of human, each theoretically fixed in a certain phenotypic expression, or at least stable enough to be knowable at neurobiological and genetic levels. Yet, in practice there is an instability about this categorical scheme. At certain stages of knowledge production, this distinction is operationalized perfunctorily, foregrounding the necessity of diametrically distinct types of research participants—"antisocial and normal," or "psychopathic and control," groups. In other phases, however, especially when it comes to potential applications or ethical imports of neurobiological substrates for violence, these categorical demarcations are ostensibly collapsed. Research groupings are reenvisioned as risk calculations that seem to blur categorical distinction in favor of an unspecified range of vulnerability. This means that the program operates through a sense of productivity in uncertainty, an unsolved tension pertaining to the ambiguity of these vital categories, which researchers nevertheless accommodate because of the indispensable empirical value that this system supposedly adds to the production of scientific knowledge.[37] Therefore, certain old ideas are relied upon as epistemological principles to support and justify the current rendition of the program, which allows neuroscientists to reject the program's deterministic or eugenic past while also discreetly preserving specific inquiries, methodologies, and ontological principles from previous eras.

Furthermore, we cannot understand the critical function or work of the program's history without considering how researchers frame today's science as a natural rebuttal to biological determinism. Neuroscientists' argument that the program's contemporary revised ontological position—that the biological and the environmental/social (biosocial) are key to understanding the roots of violence—makes the neuroscience of violence a worthwhile scientific and biomedical venture, and an important social investment. In *The Biology of Violence*, neuroscientist Deborah Niehoff argues that "critics may be fighting the same old battles, but the world itself has changed."[38] Niehoff's statement suggests that today's researchers are no longer troubled with such criticism, as the phrase "same old battles" is used in reference to controversy tied to biological determinism. The program's avowal to take the social seriously presents an interesting challenge for critics, who continue to argue that the program threatens to undermine the value of social explanations for violence. Biological determinism underpins a "slippery slope" reasoning by critics of the program. They contend that no matter the intent, biological interpretations of violence can, and undoubtedly will, be interpreted as scientific validation of a life destined for violence. This position, in large part, supports their suspicion that the program reinforces racism, sexism, and general social inequality, further marginalizes individuals labeled antisocial, psychopathic, or criminal, and justifies social control through medicalized knowledges and technical practices. Yet, where critics see the potential return of biological determinism, Niehoff and other researchers see misplaced fears and misunderstandings about the program's transformation through the mind and brain sciences. The truth, however, is somewhere in between.

Neuroscientists today reject deterministic and, as we will see, fixed understandings of biology and violence that once were considered principal components of biocriminological theories. In turn, they suggest that the violent brain construct is a more promising biomedical understanding of violence, eliminating the need to emphasize crime and criminals directly. It is important to note again that this "new generation of scientists" is composed primarily of psychologists and neuropsychologists, and that most do not have criminological training or see themselves first as researchers of crime. Moreover, they assert that the violent brain framework illustrates a social, or biosocial, representation of violence, which affords the opportunity to capture, redefine, and better "quantify things"—specifically social "things" like the environment or maltreatment, which are now understood as co-constitutive factors with biology in the etiology of violence. Thus, the biosocial rebranding of violence as a neurobiological disorder essentially incorporates and re-centers the program's most contentious implication, an apparent undermining of "the social."

Contemporary neuroscience rejects "prewired" brain arguments in favor of a "social brain," or "biosocial brain," position; thus, the brain is thought to be profoundly social by nature.[39] Accordingly, neuroscientists studying violence now contend that "if any entity deserves greater voice in the ongoing debate about violence, it is the brain. . . . It redefines violence as a developmental process rather than a character defect or an economic outcome, charting the impact of the environment on the nervous system, as well as the influence of the nervous system on the individual's response to the environment."[40] Neuroscientists defend this position by suggesting that neurobiological models have an arguably intrinsic attentiveness to the social. However, development of the power to visualize the impacts of the social through a language of brain signaling is a process that "transforms external determinants of health into internal ones."[41] The violent brain model, therefore, exemplifies a key aspect of this "regime of truth." Its role is to bind together larger social and psychological understandings, incorporating seemingly the most vital causes of such behaviors, and then remaking and reshaping these explanations into a presumably coherent, biomedically useful, and supposedly neutral reality of violence. This perspective has allowed today's researchers to wield a certain amount of authority over both past biocriminology knowledges and even sociological or anthropological theories of violence that are seen as antiquated and/or incomplete. Thus, the violent brain model has been reconceptualized and rationalized as *the* true empirical conduit to the social.

There has not been enough scrutiny about how well this model of violence meaningfully captures social experiences and actions. We must ask whether neuroscientific acknowledgment of violence as socially influenced biomedical disorder is sufficient to capture the powerful and ever shifting social dynamics that affect a society's recognition of and responses to violent behavior. This is imperative to the larger conversation about the progress of the program because these new knowledges are meant to augment, if not replace, existing social logics of violence in other social worlds—most importantly the criminal justice and policing systems. Neuroscientists are not often challenged to explain exactly how these seemingly universal neurobiological knowledges will be translated into socially and ethically productive interventions or policies that will take seriously, and not further harm, diverse groups of social bodies.

Many marginalized social groups are often already envisioned through powerful discourses of violence, and consequently managed through state-sanctioned policies that emphasize apparently inherent characteristics of "dangerousness," "illegality," "extremism," or "terror." At this point, then, it is more than rational for the public to be cautious that categorizing someone as neurobiologically susceptible to violence will be interpreted, correctly or not, as objective medical evidence of that person's culpability for criminal wrongdoing or neuroscientific proof of his or her essential nature as a criminal or violent being. Contrary to Niehoff's hopes, then, the embattled research program has not necessarily transcended the "same old battles," but is tightly tethered to them and likely will invite new controversies through this limited biomedicalized model of violence and the brain.

RISK-THINKING AND RISKY BRAINS

The conviction that neuroscientists imbue in the violent brain model—the ability to see our neurobiological underpinnings of violence, predict our antisocial mentalities, and possibly heal our criminal tendencies—is materialized through the making, manipulation, and service of this brain type. To the untrained eye, the construct of the violent brain—more specifically the produced images of this model—could easily be mistaken for, or read as, the "schizophrenic brain," "the addict brain," "the female brain," or even "the normal brain." Specialized access, knowledge, and methodologies are required to prevent such slippages, so that neuroscientists will know how to capture brain data, interpret it, and then meticulously arrange it in the correct patterns of warm and contrasting hues that make up a brain scan. However, the product is much more than a "picture" of a violent brain. This neurobiologic model of behavior highlights how the brain is continually reimagined as a technology itself. That is, the brain has been transformed into a site of knowing and intervention, where both new and old questions about the meaning, causation, and worth of violence can be unlocked. Neuroscientists' belief in the brain, then, does more than just assist other theories of violence; it becomes a perpetually malleable site of investigation, management, and imagination of risk.

Readjusting the program's focus to would-be criminals, neuroscientists have embraced and expanded the use of "risk-thinking," aiming to show their audiences in vibrant imagery who *could be* violent, rather than who *was* or *is* violent. Rose tells us that risk-thinking "denotes a family of ways of thinking and acting that involve calculations about probable futures in the present followed by interventions into the present in order to control that potential future."[42] Moreover, sociologist Robert Castel convincingly argues that the focus of psychological practices has shifted from "dangerousness to risk."[43] According to Castel, emphasis on an individual's inherent or "embodied" characteristic, dangerousness, was overwhelmingly used to justify interventions and treatments by experts in the psy-sciences. However, contemporary psy-sciences have shifted away from this dependency on dangerousness, and now have put their faith in evaluations that privilege "objective accumulation of facts." This new logic prioritizes measures outside of the individual, including lived space, social engagements, and public records, which can be collected and then tallied into an "objective" calculation of *risk*. The shift to risk means that experts no longer have to rely on individual evaluations to determine if people are a danger to society or themselves, since being determined at-risk through a risk assessment is enough to trigger the need for intervention. In this way, the program's new focus on propensity for crime may be understood as a shift that "dissolve[d] the notion of a *subject* or concrete individual, and put it in its place a combination of *factors*, factors of risk."[44]

Neuroscientific attempts to visibly outline and prove "probable futures" are indispensable elements of the program today. Here, the key concern about the violent brain framework goes beyond a biomedical challenge to free will or criminal responsibility, and instead is observed in the emergence of a different kind of violent being, "the susceptible individual."[45] Although this concept will be taken up later in the book, it is critical to note here its importance, especially the way the violent brain model can transform and rearticulate assumptions about human nature, identity, and sociality.[46] On the one hand, this model of violence invites an "objective self-fashioning," an idealized sense of worth, health, and overall "personhood,"[47] which neuroscientists framed as a potential way for susceptible individuals to know and understand their risk, to come to terms with their increased possibility to behave violently, and to potentially avoid these risks. On the other hand, the violent brain model is entrenched within existing, yet unacknowledged, sociocultural discourses, and therefore, susceptible individuals are also born through normative ideas, which can effortlessly reconstitute existing notions of difference, power, and social worth that are already entwined with social understandings of violence.

By illuminating the discursive role of risk, this book offers two interrelated observations. First, there is a need to rethink, or at least problematize, how the seemingly totalizing shift in psychological discourse from dangerousness to risk affects the translation of knowledge. That is, in order to truly assess the social implications of this new science, students of governmentality must engage with the ways that dangerousness may perform a significant function when it comes to the public's consumption and use of these knowledges of risk. Anthropologist Didier Fassin recommends that we emphasize the relations of power that operate at the levels outside the purview of population-based analytics, at the level of identity and social experiences at the margins of society.[48] Thus we may need to rethink, and unpack, what types of social influences count as risk factors for violence in the first place, and especially how existing racial, socioeconomic, and gendered life chances are encoded, and read through, these seemingly benign measures. "The fact is, risk today has collapsed into prior criminal history," argues legal scholar Bernard Harcourt, "and prior criminal history has become a proxy for race."[49]

Stratified social hierarchies challenge a uniform conception or singular expectation of the susceptible individual. Neurobiological knowledges of violence are made through and informed by the social contingencies that help produce different kinds of susceptible individuals. Thus, I call for greater attention to the unique function of conviction, how faith in "picturing personhood," unlocking the true neurobiological quality of the criminal, is allowing for new readings of "life itself," but also obscuring the way that such knowledges will likely help perpetuate devastating discourses of violence *and* safety in society.[50]

Therefore, and secondly, I argue that the violent brain model is a normative framework. Stepping back a bit, consider that neuroscientific research on violence seems to suggest that it is both specific enough to show us the underpinnings of violence in seemingly discrete biomedical populations of antisocial and criminal persons, and also malleable enough to detect hidden risk for violent behavior in general populations. Therefore, the violent brain construct operates through a *normative* valence, in that it proposes a vision of what an appropriate understanding of violence "ought to be" in order to make it usable to study via neuroscientific practices. Moreover, it has a *normalizing* imperative in the sense that the target is not simply the quintessentially antisocial individual, but essentially any person diagnosed, or "fitted," with a risky neurobiological profile. *Conviction* sheds light on the way this model helps reconstitute existing conditions of life by demonstrating where and how neuroscientific engagement with the social is anemic, dull, and overall normative. Yet, "[t]he political function of the term *normal* structures hierarchy while masking exclusion through the projection of illusionary objective norms."[51] For philosopher Joy James, this means that some bodies are situated outside of prescribed ideologies of normality, and therefore, are always already subjected to violent forms of correction and punishment by virtue of their racialized and gendered positionalities. Thus, this book demonstrates that the greatest weakness of the research program is an extraordinary inability to truly handle, discern, and conceptualize complex sociocultural dynamics, chiefly inequality.

By tracing sociocultural assumptions and expectations built into the making and practices of the violent brain construct, *Conviction* goes beyond traditional and broadly applied critiques of biological determinism, to parse and anticipate new social and ethical consequences of the biology of violence. I do not question the authenticity of the program's shift toward biosocial dimensions; it is clear that today's researchers have carved out an increasing advantageous epistemological space for social and environmental factors. Similarly, there is an importance to thinking more complexly about the intricate and interlocked intersections between biology and sociocultural factors. I do question, however, the usefulness of this framework for highly socialized and uniquely politicized behaviors like violence or crime. This leads me to ask: What exactly does the program's progress, supposedly afforded through better measures and technologies, mean for the lives of groups of individuals whose social experiences are left out of these models? Thus we must think critically about the bodies that are undertheorized or overlooked in this framework, the brains of individuals that do not fit neatly into this logic. These are the embodied experiences that are seemingly too complex to fully comprehend in neurobiological reasoning as it stands today, yet they will nevertheless be rendered as objectively knowable and predictable "cerebral subjects" for courtrooms, parole boards, or classrooms.

READING CONVICTION

The book is divided into two parts. Part I: "The Making of the Violent Brain" (Chapters 1–3) and Part II: "The Unmaking of the Violent Brain" (Chapters 4–7). Part I provides analysis of the vital theoretical and technical aspects of the science, with the goal of outlining the social practices that appear invisible or become "lost" in the development of the violent brain framework. Specifically, I situate this section around the *management of uncertainty*. As the subtitle indicates, chapters in this section trace the production of the violent brain in research, elucidating the technical, cultural, and social assumptions that help to preserve some sense of scientific objectivity, and illustrating how neuroscientists negotiate and construct a sense of empirical certitude through technologically assisted engagements with the brain. The making of the violent brain also draws attention to the relationship between neuroscientists' work toward certitude and an ever expanding fluidity in the idea of risk-thinking. Part I of *Conviction* shows that the production of neurobiological knowledges of violence simultaneously shapes neuroscientific expectations of both "violent" *and* "normal" behaviors *and* brains.

A fundamental critique of the research program rests on the idea that violence is socially constructed, and therefore cannot be reliably understood through a strict biological framework. Chapter 2 details the malleable and precarious use of diagnostic and classificatory systems to medicalize, identify, and sort bodies for neuroscientific research on violence, which is then used to reframe violence into a medical model of antisocial behavior along a spectrum of biomedical risk. The use of a "medical model" of violence is not new. The revised biomedicalized version of violence presented here, however, gains its scientific credence through the fusion of old classificatory systems with new technical tools, which allow neuroscientists to assemble a medical definition of violence that presumably warrants the neurobiological study of such behaviors, what I call the "fitting" process.

Brain scans, the premier technological product of scanning, are the focus of Chapter 3. Neuroscientific imaging technologies have allowed researchers to "see" the brain's morphology and track its performance. In turn, researchers of violence have used these tools to help identify biomedically "abnormal" brain architecture thought to increase the risk for violence. The violent brain construct, however, is not just a way to visualize the brains of potential criminals; implicitly it outlines the empirical boundaries for the brains of normal or well-behaved populations too. Researchers' ability to visualize risk in terms of brain structure and function, therefore, expands the power of the program's epistemic culture of risk-thinking. Furthermore, Chapter 3 demonstrates that imaging technologies offer an unquestioned cultural and scientific authority, which tends to obscure imprecise measurements, experimental uncertainties, and ethical questions that lie at the heart of the research.

If "making" the violent brain centers on the management of uncertainty, and how neuroscientists ostensibly work against the social, then its "unmaking" concerns techniques of anticipation,[52] in particular how neuroscientists attempt to work with, appreciate, and incorporate the social into models of violent behavior. The violent brain model moved the science into a better position to utilize social causes, but this turn has also left researchers ill-equipped to navigate complex sociocultural circumstances that relentlessly structure and dictate how we enact, know, and manage violence. Yet, when neuroscientists blur the lines between "violently at-risk" brain function and "normal" brain function, they are also increasing the possibilities for new sociopolitical ramifications, such as revised surveillance tactics that will empower individuals, and the state, help manage risky brains. Each chapter in Part II makes clear that the violent brain model is intrinsically replete with insufficient considerations of social dynamics. The results here point to a limiting way in which the "social" is conceptualized and operationalized in such models, which, I argue, has detrimental impacts on the ability to account for the social, ethical, and political implications of the science. The most critical drawback is the inability of neuroscientists to fully capture social experiences, especially disparate social conditions that untimely dictate exposure to contingent and unequal life chances; hence, essential risk factors of violent or criminal behaviors.

Chapter 4 turns to genetic knowledges of violence and their relationship to the brain. A closer look at contemporary genetic claims about violence reveals an inseparable connection to the brain sciences. Genes that have been linked to violent behaviors are said to moderate the brain's ability to regulate conduct. More specifically, they are "neurogenetic" biomarkers thought to raise an individual's risk for personality disorders, and hence increase the propensity for violent or antisocial behavior. It is more appropriate, therefore, to consider neuroscientific and genetic approaches to violence as sociotechnical practices—instead of distinct disciplinary groupings—united under a neurobiological *thought-style* of violence. Genetic, specifically gene x environment interaction (GxE), research is key to the program's designated turn away from biological determinism. However, the measurement and conceptualization of the "environment" in these approaches can discursively operate to reify the authority of the biological. Put plainly, these models of violence often reinforce the social and the environment as *secondary* to the biological, which undermines or devalues the dynamic influences of social factors. I question whether neuroscientists' reflexivity toward the causes of violent behavior, particularly measuring some factor of "environment," fully captures or includes meaningful social experiences. Thus, limitations of the violent brain model are inhibiting the "(bio)sociological imagination" that neuroscientists seek to exhibit.[53]

Race, and especially its mistaken meaning as a biological reality, has been imperative to the biology of violence since its formal inception as a "scientific" discipline. The neuroscience literature on violence bares a conspicuous absence of any mention of race, and some neuroscientists, like many other behavioral scientists, have adopted a "race-neutral" approach to help avoid backlash due to finding or reporting racial differences in their results. However, this move away from race has severely limited the ability of this model to acknowledge and deal with the *effects* of race; the dynamic and often embedded ways in which the oppressive realities of systemic inequality and the discursive articulations of prejudicial ideology structure the way a society constructs, knows, and deals with racially marginalized groups. Chapter 5 interrogates the haunting "absent presence of race," and I argue that the violent brain model has actually (re)produced a color-blind logic in the biology of violence.[54] This has allowed researchers to generate a biological understanding of violence seemingly without fear of backlash, yet it has also has nullified their ability to address the "writing of race into crime."[55] That is, the concurrent and discursive ways in which social logics of violence rely on race being criminalized and crime being racialized, as a preeminent function of law and order and a key element in the spectacle of public safety endorsed by governmental bodies.

Chapter 6 considers the potential interventions onto and into the violent brain construct that primarily function as a means to elucidate risk for violence. The salience of this type of risk modeling, then, is better captured as a "therapeutic promise," which rebuffs the allure of an immediate cure for violence and instead envisions prospective treatment options for behavioral risk in the near future.[56] The benefit of the violent brain model is that it often places greater emphasis on improving social conditions to address the brain risk for violence. Yet, the therapeutic promise coincidentally points to environmental change *and* places acute fixation on individual optimization, as a self-centered expectation of at-risk individuals to work upon themselves. Thus, Chapter 6 points to the development of new imaginaries of neurobiological risk, in which neuroscientists chase an ultimate goal of biomedical prediction, a neuro-speculative "mind reading." Consequently, neuro-prediction presents as a more informative way to calculate and treat risk; however, this practice of scientific anticipation, consequently, expands target populations toward normal individuals at younger and healthier stages of life. The therapeutic promise attached to the violent brain construct raises critical questions about the role of the state, principally criminal justice institutions, in neuroscientific solutions for violence. As these knowledges travel beyond the lab, they can help to inconspicuously authorize new corporeal surveillance tactics that may bolster already problematic law enforcement policies through a guise of social wellness and safety.

Conviction concludes with Chapter 7, in which I propose the need to refocus attention on the *new* uncertainties, slippages, and reductionisms surrendered in the contemporary (un)making of the neurobiological subject.[57] Rather than identifying the violent brain model as a refashioned mechanism of biological determinism, I argue that this construct—its social potential, and empirical value for the research program—is more aptly understood through the way it empowers practices of *reading, forgetting, and envisioning* the social, or a socialness, of violence. Biological determinism is not necessarily an inconsequential factor for the violent brain. Instead, this framework performs a slightly different kind of fixing. The violent brain model is not about one's predestined fate—i.e., a life of crime—but a more obscure and equally troubling alignment of the entangled bonds between the body and sociality, which seek to "prove" the best, or more complete, way to understand and effectively treat violence. The book's concluding chapter cautions that these neuro-knowledges of violence may further preserve seemingly static hierarchies of subjectivity, not through old bio-deterministic means, but through the sheer omission of lived experiences, a normative inattention to lives, and inability of this neuro-technique to seriously challenge racialized, marginalized, and "inferiorized" practices that construct the "abnormal" social behaviors we recognized as violent, antisocial, criminal, and that are embodied through the human beings critical to this inquiry.[58]

2 | FINDING THE "FIT"

THE UNDERPINNINGS OF TODAY'S brain-based under-
standing of violence can be traced back, at least in part, to the expansion
of biocriminology during the Weimar period in Germany.[1] As notions of
the "born criminal" were falling out of favor, themselves highly influenced
by phrenological and evolutionary arguments of the nineteenth century,
German biocriminology was debating the best way to move forward, which
yielded different factions in disagreement about the epistemological underpinnings or applications for the research program. The shifts taking place
during this period foreshadowed the gradual dispersal of the research program by the end of World War II, and its piecemeal reclamation, and eventual
return, into more-legitimate psy-disciplines in Europe and the United States
by the mid-1960s. Through these latter transformations, violent and criminal
behaviors were redefined as biomedical entities and therefore designated
suitable for biological study.[2]

University of London psychologist Hans J. Eysenck's 1964 publication,
Crime and Personality, was the first notable theory on the biology of violence after World War II. Capturing the convoluted reception and lasting
significance of *Crime and Personality*, historian Nicole Rafter argues that it
was "the publication that first reinserted a biological voice into the chorus
of sociological explanations, sounding a theme that became steadily louder
over the following decades."[3] Eysenck's argument focused on two points: first,

personality, specifically learning and conditioning, was the basis of crime; and second, personality was rooted in biology.[4] He relied on more-traditional psychological research to make his argument that personality was related to crime, but the second part of the thesis used Ivan Pavlov's then novel work on conditioning and new revelations from hereditary research on violence.[5] Following Eysenck's lead, a new wave of biological-based research on violence emerged, launching the medicalization era of the program.[6]

By the 1970s, dramatic increases in crime rates in the United States provided an opening for the research program to regain its footing. During this period, the reallocation of resources to policing and legal arenas led to political and financial support for medically driven (via psychology) interventions to combat rising crime rates.[7] The larger social implications of this move worried many critics, already skeptical of the promises that biological researchers made, given the notorious history of the field. They feared that the "unholy alliance"[8] between medicine and law enforcement would divert attention from what they saw as more-promising social or political interventions. Indeed, the medicalization of violence, some argued, would restructure ideas about, and dictate the terms of, criminal accountability, and ultimately expand the authoritative role of the state through a more palatable rhetoric of public health and medical care.[9]

The most direct way to think about medicalization is to consider how a concept, behavior, or trait that is usually defined outside of medical terms, falls under the purview of medical authority. With regard to violence and crime, medicalization shifts interests from one social world (legal) to another (medical). Importantly, this shift redefines the behaviors or traits in question. In response, critics of medicalization, like sociologists Peter Conrad and Joseph Schneider, reiterated that such behaviors do not represent objective and/or static understandings of "unacceptable" behavior. Rather, our understandings of these behaviors derive from socially constructed meanings that are always contingent on societal interactions, politics, institutions, and time.[10] Conrad and Schneider's argument also shows that the shift from sociolegal meaning to medical terminology does not guarantee the materialization of objective understandings for the types of traits, actions, or feelings that are recognized as violence. Definitions of violence exist within contested spheres of power, in which labeling behavior is a political action, and therefore inherently uncertain. "The power to diagnose—that is to give names to—problematic behavior," writes neuropsychologist Stephan Chorover, "is one aspect of the power to define the limits of allowable behavioral diversity in a society. And, in any society, the power to give names and to enforce definitions is a touchstone of social control."[11]

By the late 1970s, it appeared that critics of the medicalization of violence were getting their message through to both political and lay publics. They had objected to the medicalization of violence and its promise for biomedical treatments, like psychosurgery, to "cure" violent offenders. Horrifying stories of brain lobotomies gone wrong, and the growing concern that the real aim of such procedures was to control or emaciate black populations, all but extinguished the initiative to "fix" bad brains. However, this victory against medicalization was temporary. The missteps with the medicalization of violence in the 1960s and 1970s became points of correction and reflection for contemporary researchers—rather than reasons to end the program entirely, which critics were likely aiming for.

When the neuroscience of violence emerged in the late 1980s, it marked a shift, a transformation from a medicalization of violence that was criticized primarily as state-sanctioned therapeutic *control*, to a *bio*medicalization of violence organized around a framework of anticipation and a therapeutic *promise*.[12] The biomedical meanings of violence that emerged during the medicalization period were reworked through technological assistance into genetic and neurobiological contingencies. Sociologist Adele Clarke and colleagues note that biomedicalization captures the intricately embedded relationships between the engines of medicalization and the multiplicity of "conditions of possibility" that emerged alongside the start of the molecular-ization era.[13] Essentially, biomedicalization differs from classic medicalization critiques that emphasized the practices of social control through medical expansion via the reconceptualization of the social world in medical or health terms, by focusing on the *transformations* of health, illness, and the body from the "inside out," through the rapid rise of and ever more prevalent dependence on technoscientific practices—that is, the hybrid product of science *and* technology.[14] By focusing on the increasing technoscientific influence on illness, health, *and* well-being (or what it means to be healthy), and not only on the expanding jurisdiction of medicine, biomedicalization sets out to address the influential effects of biomedicine and science on everyday "ways of knowing" and practices of "living" in society. For our purposes, however, the focus on redefining violence into a medical illness afforded through biomedicalization was essential for neuroscientists' ability to push back against critiques of the program.

VIOLENCE AS AN ILLNESS

Critiques of biological theories of violence point to social, cultural, and historical ambiguities as undeniable evidence that these behaviors are socially constructed, and therefore unexplainable through a strict biological rationale. Sociologist Troy Duster contends that imprecise understandings of violent behavior, and the uneven or interchangeable applications of descriptors like "criminal" or "delinquent," undermine scientific attempts to explain them through natural laws. According to Duster, there has been a lack of a "theoretical warrant" to investigate violence in biological terms—an inability to justify and precisely outline the set of behaviors that uniquely require attention from the biological sciences. He asks, "What is the theoretical warrant for designating certain behaviors the subject of behavioral genetics [or neurobiological explanation] while ignoring or dismissing others?"[15] In other words, given the vast spectrum of social behaviors, why has the program, as well as certain public interests, invested so much scientific capital in the study of violence? Here, I quote Duster's critique of the genetics of violence at length:

> The search for a genetic explanation for such a demonstrably variegated phenotype (criminal) requires a theoretical warrant that has never been delivered. The closest that one can come is in the abstracted notion of an "antisocial personality," but even for this abstracted version the obstacles to linking phenotypes to genotypes are huge. That is, given this demonstrably high empirical variability (sometimes arbitrary, sometimes systemic reach of the criminal justice system) in what constitutes a crime, and even more demonstrably high empirical variability in what constitutes "antisocial behavior" across social time and space, how is it possible to search for a genotype? The answer, and conclusion, provide strong reasons for deep concern.[16]

Duster illuminates an inherent contradiction in the program: If scientists are unable to firmly define the object of their exploration, then how can they propose a natural, purportedly universal, biological explanation of such traits? How are neuroscientists rationalizing the study of violent behavior if the meanings of such behavior are contextually specific and their recognition and manifestation in a society continually shift?

Researchers today acknowledge the difficulties and uncertainties that permeate this ontological condition. Literature from neuroscience and psychology suggests that researchers are still debating which behaviors matter, or should count, for their study of violence. In their review on neuroimaging and violence, Jana Bufkin and Vickie Luttrell (a criminologist and a psychologist, respectively) define violence as behaviors that violate social norms and inflict physical injury, and aggression as threatening or actual assaultive behavior toward a person or environment.[17] In reality, however, it is difficult to imagine a behavior that would violate social norms and impose physical injury *without* also being threatening or assaultive behavior. In fact, with the exception of these initial definitions, Bufkin and Luttrell use the phrase "aggression and/or violence" throughout the remainder of the review; an acknowledgment of the overlapping use of these terms in neuroimaging research. Similarly, representatives from the Aspen Neurobehavioral Conference (ANC) acknowledge the fluid application of these terms in their consensus statement on the neurobiological factors of violence.[18] Their definition of aggression is similar to that of Bufkin and Luttrell: an adaptive and intentional act that causes physical and/or mental harm. Violence, however, becomes a variation of aggression for the ANC group, which they characterize as an aggressive act that leads to unwarranted physical injury.

The difficulty in explicating clear use of these terms, and even their seemingly synonymous connotation, is not unusual. Psychiatrist Jan Volavka notes that different disciplines set their own rules about the meanings for terms like "violence" and "aggression." "*Violence*" is more often used in sociological and legal research, according to Volavka, while psychological, psychiatric, and biological researchers prefer the term "*aggression*."[19] Nevertheless, disciplinary boundaries do not really explain the interchangeable use of these terms in neurobiological research—Volavka's own book is titled *Neurobiology of Violence*, although it is presumably written as a neuropsychological text. The overwhelming majority of the neuroscientific studies I analyzed focused on standard classifications in the field, especially "antisocial behavior." Antisocial behavior is seen by some researchers as a more comprehensive concept than either violence or aggression. Psychologists Rolf Loeber and Dustin Pardini write that "violence refers to forcible robbery, attacking with intent to injure, sexual coercion, or rape; aggression, on the other hand, refers to lessor injurious acts, whereas antisocial behavior is a *general* term encompassing aggression, violence, and non-violent forms of delinquency."[20]

My use of the term "violence" throughout this book is not intended to erase these intricate differences, or to suggest that neuroscientists work with a specific or definitive description of such behaviors. Instead, I opt for this term because it seems to better capture the malleability, in terms of application, that neuroscientists have afforded this neurobiological model. That is, it seems to better capture the way neurosciences generalize and rationalize the societal purpose and worth of these knowledges. While researchers do want a scientific understanding of violence, they also seem to want such a model to speak to the everyday set of behaviors that we all "know" or recognize as violence. Thus, researchers may focus their inquiry on aggression, psychopathy, or even impulsivity as a behavioral trait; however, the potential impacts of the science are framed as a biomedical or health response to the enduring problem of violence, if not criminal violence, within society. For example, Kent Kiehl starts off his book *The Psychopath Whisperer* with a detailed description of the first time he entered a prison to study inmates.[21] The preface of *Biology of Aggression*, edited by neuroscientist Randy Nelson, begins:

> The effects of aggression and violence on people can be seen in the news media every day. Whether the story is about the mauling of a woman by an aggressive dog, students attacking their colleagues in school, workers attacking their colleagues at work, or people detonating bombs in response to their ideological beliefs, unchecked aggression and violence exact a significant toll on society.[22]

My point here is that social and ethical expectations about social behavior are an important part of the way this science perceives its object of study, which is then rearticulated, reconstituted, and sharpened through its production and potential use. "Scientific theories are work, not disembodied ideas," states sociologist Susan L. Star. "That is, people do not unearth facts—they assemble, array, propose, and defend them from their situations."[23]

Getting back to Duster's question about theoretical warrant, neuroscientists frame violent acts as characteristics or traits of a special class of psychological disorders outlined in *Diagnostic and Statistical Manual of Mental Disorders* (*DSM*) (the diagnostic handbook of the American Psychiatric

Association).[24] This medicalized perspective is keenly aimed at the brains of clinical populations. That is, this research operates, generally, through two interrelated steps. First, diagnosis of a personality disorder, ascertained through criteria outlined in *DSM* and other psychological screening checklists, scales, and questionnaires.[25] Next, researchers use experimental testing to illuminate brain region(s) that are likely involved with the disorder in question. We can think about prevalent use of *DSM* classifications, then, as a proxy way for researchers to outline the targeted behavior(s) of their research. Seemingly, the research focus is on the bond between certain personality disorders and violence (or aggression). In other words, researchers indicate that they are interested in violence, actually the risk for violence, to understand the function of these mental disorders or an individual's risk for them in the future.

The importance of this biomedical description is that it presumably provides an experimental field through which biology is more justified. Health problems, in this rationale, should require answers that are, at least principally, focused on biomedical or biological causation. The justification goes more or less like this: If violence can be reframed as a biomedical symptom for medical conditions, then it would seem prudent to consider the neurobiological roots of such a symptom. That is, by shifting the program's focus to the risk of particular psychological disorders, a neurobiological investigation is not only warranted but seemingly necessary. *DSM* classifications, in theory, provide a more reliable and appropriate rubric to approach violence than penal descriptors like "criminal" or "murderer," sociolegal concepts that neuroscientists consider less relevant for scientific inquiry.[26] However, the *DSM* has its own sociocultural import and taxonomic complexities that render its applicability in scientific research just as problematic and uncertain as criminal justice labels.[27] And, as we will see in Chapter 3, this epistemological framework requires additional work, specifically through the assistance of other technologies, in order to truly actualize; and even then the model still suffers fundamental problems. Thus, the biomedicalization of violence alone is not enough to overcome Duster's criticism.

"FITTING" VIOLENCE INTO CLINICAL DIAGNOSTICS

Along with the debates with outside critics, neuroscientists also have disagreements within the program. There are important differences within the field regarding the way researchers think about the utility of neuroscience research on violence, which stems from deeper ontological differences in the way the framing of violence is differentially operationalized in the research. For most, the goal of this research is to elucidate neurobiological risk factors for personality disorders related to violent behavior. For others, however, like neuropsychologist Adrian Raine, this biomedicalized framework could be extended to other forms of violence; that is, abnormal or damaged brains may be a causal factor for all criminal behaviors.

Raine's importance to the development and achievement of the neuroscience of violence cannot be overstated. He is arguably the most recognizable neuropsychologist studying violence. Raine pioneered the first set of neuroimaging studies on violence during the 1990s, as discussed in Chapter 3, and later coined the term "neurocriminology," as a distinct subfield devoted to brain research on violence. However, Raine is also unique in other ways. He works in the University of Pennsylvania's criminology department as well as holding appointments in psychiatry and psychology; therefore he is an essential asset for the program as it continues to branch out and rework other fields like biosocial criminology.[28] However, some other neuroscientists have regarded the use of neuroscience as a supplement to general theory crime as inappropriate and a bit provocative.

There is a key tension between the various actors in the program. While Raine views a "broken brain" as a basis for *any* crime, other neuropsychologists have tried to adhere more strictly to a biomedical understanding of antisocial behavior. This position was highlighted during my interview with Dr. Lewis. Throughout our conversation, Dr. Lewis emphasized the salience of the ontological tension in the program, which can be summed up in this passionate response:

> Researchers need to be assessing and quantifying behaviors and traits and not just say that they want to study violence in general. If it's a biological trait, a person will be violent at home, at work, at school, with their family, with friends. Whereas crime per se is very much a social problem. It's miscarriage of justice and science to try to treat somebody who commits a single crime as a violent individual. There are a million different reasons why people are violent, which means there's a million different brain neurons that were engaged differently. . . . My point is, you need to be a *good* psychologist.[29]

Raine, I assume, would agree that "there are a million different reasons why people are violent." However, his work also implies that it may be too presumptuous to dismiss a brain understanding of general crime. Dr. Lewis, on the other hand, is less convinced that neurobiological explanations can provide enough useful information for non-pathological criminal or violent behavior. For this researcher, being a "good psychologist" implies a more meticulous approach to the violent behavior, one that stays within the bounds of clinically explainable tendencies for such acts.

Struggles with this "unstable referent," then, are a core feature of the program, and the manner in which neuroscientists try to resolve, or at least minimize, this problem helps to illuminate the social nature that underpins neurobiological research on violence.[30] Yet in some important areas of this work, the two sides seem to overlap. When it comes to questions about developing the right presentation, or biomedical framing, for violence, these differences in ontological viewpoints have not impeded the production of knowledge.[31] I am suggesting that before neuroscientists begin their studies, they must first perform work to "(re)frame" violent behavior(s) into suitable scientific commodities that warrant biomedical and technological probing. In this process, classificatory uncertainty at times can work as an asset, since the malleability of these descriptive meanings and criteria for personality disorders, and therefore violence, can be more easily shaped to work within neurobiological framework; I call this work *fitting*.

In this biomedical framing, the meaning of violent behavior goes beyond proving or disproving the existence of a psychopathology (i.e., a mental illness or disorder). Rather, fitting reflects a practice that considers the wide variety of diagnostic criteria for mental disorder and tries to extract the most appropriate neuropsychological explanation for violent and aggressive behavioral tendencies. As captured by Raine in his book *The Psychopathology of Crime*, "although no single definition clearly delineates psychopathology, the many definitions, when taken together, create a general 'gestalt' or picture of what constitutes a psychopathology. . . . *The key question is whether these definitions provide any degree of 'fit' to criminal behavior.*"[32] Neuroscientists, then, are actively shaping diagnostic possibilities by working through a sense of fluidity that is supposedly allowed from biomedical understandings of violence. The goal here is not necessarily to know or define what violence is, but to leverage the ways in which specific ways to recognize, count, and discern "violence" thus hold these items in a coordinated and steady fashion long enough to produce a neurobiological account of mental illness.

Fitting operates as a complex, multi-sided series of ongoing negotiations among diagnostic criteria, technological innovation, and scientific expertise. In other words, it provides an epistemological space where classification and standardization converge. If classifications represent a way of sorting and ordering groups, standards are the subtle, often invisible, rules of governance that help achieve this system over multiple sites and uses.[33] Standardization allows researchers to use classificatory protocols with confidence, yet these rules of practices often accentuate the intrinsic heterogeneity and uncertainty in classification schemas, which then force researchers to reformulate or negotiate how to read or enact standards in order to efficiently employ them in research.

This process works with, and not against, definitional variabilities. It implicitly places two categorical disputes in exchange with each other, the classificatory slippages endemic in taxonomies of psychopathology and the definitional difficulties emblematic of terminologies for violence. What emerges, or what is hoped for, is that criminal and violent behaviors are situated, or likened to, the definitional and operational terrain of mental disorders, and that such a framework remains stable, or steady enough, to endure the experimental stage of research. However, as sociologist Martyn Pickersgill posits, "uncertainties endure—in part—precisely because of attempts to build consensus regarding the ontology of antisociality through biomedical means."[34] Close attention to the fitting process helps illuminate such instabilities in early stages of this research. It demonstrates the inevitable necessity to manage continual uncertainties in order to perform a science of violence. Below, I outline the several stages of this process of fitting: recruitment of study groups, classification/diagnosis practices, quantifying the traits of violence, and the reading of qualification of these measures. In practice, this is not a stepwise process, but these practices are dependent on one another, and that becomes even more important to help neuroscientists in the next stage of the science: detecting these abnormal brain profiles under the scanner.

RECRUITMENT: "ACCESS TO THE IMPORTANT POPULATIONS"

Even though neuroscientists want to limit their focus to "clinically" violent groups, recruitment practices often lead neuroscientists to offender and incarcerated populations that are, at least partly, marked by socially constructed legal identities (i.e., murderer, felon, inmate, criminal). For example, U.S.-based researchers must often find a way into prisons or jails in order to do some of their work. "Individuals with antisocial personality disorder, or psychopathic personality disorder, end up getting in quite a bit of trouble," Dr. Garrett stated in our interview; hence "about fifteen percent of prison populations will meet criteria for psychopathy, which is about fifteen times greater than the one percent estimate in the general population." Similarly, neurologist Pamela Blake and cognitive neuroscientist Jordan Grafman write that neurobiological violence research is interested in those "violent and aggressive individuals [that] are repeat offenders."[35] However, external and ethical constraints have led many neuroscientists to recruit participants from the general public. Neuropsychiatrist Dr. Hollowell addressed this point in our interview. As Dr. Hollowell stated, studies from the Hollowell Lab

> have always been in either, you know, sort of standard research populations or community populations. So, they are not [individuals] with severely rough personality disorders, but they definitely had aggression and personality problems. We would run ads that would say things like, "Anger: can you keep it from getting into trouble?" And so, people coming in were self-identified as having problems with anger and aggression. They're community subjects in the sense that they're coming from the community. They're not like an epidemiological sample that we pulled in a random sort of way. They're a sort of self-identified collection.

The idea that individuals are simply self-selecting downplays the additional work that this lab puts into fitting. Self-identifying participants still go through the diagnostic assessments, so they are not automatically "participants" just because they answered the ad. In our conversation, Dr. Jones expanded on the relationships between advertising and screening practices for study recruitment:

> We advertise for people who deal with anger, who experience a lot of anger or are quick to blow off their steam, and that's how we advertise. We advertise in newspapers or in flyers that we hang in specific target areas, like bars and places like that where people drink a lot of alcohol, and some of them have issues with self-control so when they drink. And then they call us, and we screen them carefully. And the ones who would

qualify for IED, for intermittent explosive disorder, or for a sub-threshold diagnosis of IED, come to our labs, and then we—they sign the consent form, and they go through all the procedures. The procedures are behavioral, neuropsychological. We have EEG. We have brain imaging, fMRI, and of course extensive psychiatric interviewing. And we take their blood for DNA analysis.

Both researchers' procedures demonstrate how neuroscientists must "make" their populations. This process starts in the development of advertising and recruitment materials and is further realized through biomedical screening means once its constituents enter the lab. Unlike Dr. Hollowell, however, Dr. Jones characterizes participants as a "clinical sample," not a "community" one, although both labs seem to use very similar methods, ones that Dr. Hollowell explicitly described as not being epidemiological or standard random samples of individuals. One explanation for this subtle difference in terms may speak to the way that the two neuroscientists think about the application of this model. That is, for Dr. Jones the substitution of "community" for "clinical" may signal that their position aligns closer with Dr. Lewis's advice to focus neuroscientific research on clear, identifiable, biological traits of violence, or at least a concerted attention to be a "good psychologist."

For other neuroscientists, with study population characteristics that differ, accessibility and logistical difficulties often hinder access to needed populations. This speaks to the intricacies of "recruitmentology," what sociologist Steven Epstein defines as the study of "evaluating the efficacy of various social, cultural, psychological, technological, and economic means of convincing people, *especially members of 'hard-to-recruit populations'* that they want to become, and remain, human subjects."[36] "Pragmatically, studying adults with psychopathic traits is very difficult for brain imaging research. Recruitment-wise, it's almost impossible," says interviewee Dr. Smith. Similarly, Dr. Jones also noted that "so many people do this research and they don't really have access to the important populations. So, you have Kent Kiehl, you have this mobile MRI. These are the things that really facilitate the research and research integration."

Neuropsychologist Kent Kiehl is one researcher who has been able to access the important population, prisoners. Incarcerated individuals are characterized as a vulnerable population because researchers have inflicted ethical abuses toward this group in the past and because their confinement status can unduly influence their ability to consent for research participation. Thus, while access to prisoners can be difficult for any researcher, the task is even more challenging for neuroscientists, who also want to scan their brains. However, Kiehl's "mobile MRI" creates a new path for those with the means to access this "important population." Even before neuroimaging takes place, there is a particular "scientific capital" that comes along with the means to invest in technological innovation.[37]

Kiehl, like Raine, is well known for his lectures and presentations to audiences all around the country. He has gained fame through interviews on outlets like the *Today Show* and the PBS documentary *Brains on Trial* and has also helped form MINDSET, a consulting group that advises universities and pharmaceutical companies on neuroimaging techniques, equipment, and analysis, and assists lawyers and judges about the best practices, and potential misuses, of neuroscientific data in criminal courts. Kiehl's public recognition is driven in part by his extant research and publication record, which itself is a direct result of his ability to circumvent problems of accessibility to incarcerated populations with his mobile MRI machine.

In his book *The Psychopath Whisperer*, Kiehl recalls that his interest in obtaining a mobile MRI machine derived, somewhat ironically, from his near accident with a trucker hauling one. Kiehl would later convince the driver to allow him to take a look inside the trailer. Describing the incident, Kiehl writes:

> To my right was a door that contained all the hardware that ran the MRI. The middle room, where I was standing, was a long, narrow control room with a desk and chair. To my left was a door with a window next to it. I could see the MRI at the far rear of the trailer—-positioned right in the middle of two oddly spaced axles balancing the weights, I assumed. . . . [T]he MRI was not the type or quality that we needed for our research, but it planted a seed in my brain. . . . I thanked the driver and sat there in my Toyota as he pulled away. *Someday*, I thought.[38]

Kiehl would later leave his position at Yale University's School of Medicine for the University of New Mexico, after the southwestern school offered him a position that included a mobile MRI. He also negotiated entrée into several New Mexico prisons, with the help of the university and the governor's office.

Prison officials were eager to participate in his studies, according to Kiehl, though the facilitation of this partnership between neuroscience and criminal justice required a substantial amount of coordination and prep work.

A mobile MRI machine meant that Kiehl could bypass many of the recruitment barriers that affected his colleagues. Indeed, at the end of his first year, without the necessity of sharing time and access to the scanner like others in traditional university settings, Kiehl's lab scanned more than five hundred inmates—an impressive number given that typical sample sizes for imaging studies on violence range from ten to fifteen individuals.[39] Kiehl's use of a mobile MRI demonstrates how socioeconomic resources and social capital are entangled with, and help moderate, the elastic relationships between fitting and recruitmentology.[40]

CLASSIFICATIONS: THE ABNORMAL WITHIN THE ABNORMAL

Once researchers gain access to study populations, they must then begin to screen these populations. This step returns the conversation to definitional disputes about the meaning of violence and its biomedical import. When asked to talk about what made him interested in this research, Dr. Lewis told me that his interest in the neuroscience of violence arose from a curiosity about the "highest risk, hardest to study kind of individuals":

> I'm less interested in the—not disinterested, but less interested—in the study of just crime per se, or violence per se. . . . My work specifically focuses on the small subset of individuals that we identify as psychopaths. How to understand their brain systems and how [to] develop treatments. Specifically, for those most difficult—highest risk, hardest to study kind of individuals. The classic kind of "Hannibal Lecter" kind of person who is very different.

Researchers, therefore, are interested in these potential social threats because they are believed to exhibit an uncontrollable mental predisposition toward violence that cannot be explained by socioeconomic or cultural forces alone. Dr. Lewis's reference to the fictitious cannibal psychiatrist Hannibal Lecter captures the assumed rarity of these individuals in the larger population and the clinical fascination to *know* this unique type of criminal. Importantly, these comments also signal that a key research attribute for neuroscientists is to distinguish between regular criminals and clinical ones.

"A focus on crime, per se, is misguided from a measurement standpoint since crime is an abstract legal and social construct, not a measurable behavioral construct," writes criminologist Diana Fishbein.[41] Similarly, Dr. Lewis in our interview made a point to declare less interest in "the study of just crime per se, or violence per se." Classifications that this schema enables scientists to identify clinical forms of violence. In this sense, any meaning or measure that is thought to be a departure from standard crime, and therefore from normal brain function (variability) can imply pathology. To investigate that possibility, the most important, and maybe most obvious, tool for fitting is the *DSM*.

The *DSM* is used in neurobiological research on violence to capture clinical traits for those at highest risk for violent behavior. Diagnoses related to violence are grouped under "personality disorders" and "disruptive, impulse-control, and conduct disorders" in the *DSM*.[42] These diagnoses include antisocial personality disorder (ASPD), conduct disorder (CD), intermittent explosive disorder (IED), and oppositional defiant disorder (ODD). Two other *non-DSM* mental health classifications—psychopathy and the presence of callous-unemotional (CU) traits—are also used in neuroscience research because of their explicit link to violent behavior.[43] Conduct disorder (CD)—essentially the youth version of ASPD—and ODD are classifications primarily associated with populations under 18 years old. On the other hand, youth who exhibit what in adults would be regarded as psychopathic tendencies—chiefly a lack of both guilt and empathy for others—and display antisocial traits fall under the diagnosis callous-unemotional traits (CU).[44] Of course, a critical question here is what makes these descriptions differ from descriptions of criminal behavior. One way neuroscientists try to distinguish these clinical classifications from criminally deviant behavior is through the observation of behavioral patterns. Thus, "variability and vulnerability are treated as interchangeable constructs" in the neuroscience of violence.[45]

Fishbein's understanding of a measurable behavior is a "longstanding or *recurrent* pattern of antisocial behavior [that] is more likely due to the cumulative, developmental influence of interacting biological and environmental factors."[46] Words like "recurrent" or "repetitive" used to describe patterns of behavior also appear in diagnostic manuals. The *DSM* notes that an "essential feature of conduct disorder is a *repetitive* and *persistent pattern* of behavior in which the basic rights of others or major age-appropriate societal norms or rules are violated."[47] Psychiatrist Emil Coccaro, a leading expert on intermittent explosive disorder (IED), similarly characterizes the diagnosis as *recurring* aggressive outbursts, *repeated patterns* of verbal or physical aggression toward others or property, and/or aggressive behavior that is out of proportion to its stressors.[48] Likewise, ASPD diagnostic criteria state that it must present as "a pervasive pattern," yet only when traits are inflexible, maladaptive, and persistent, and cause significant functional impairment or subjective distress, do they constitute antisocial personality disorder."[49] The ability to measure patterns in behavior, therefore, helps to determine who should be examined, and who is suitable for study, using a neuroscientific framework.

It seems unlikely, however, that measurable patterns of behavior move the science beyond the notion of crime. Crime may be an "abstract legal and social construct," but classifications like psychopathy or antisocial behavior are relational aspects between neuro and social rationalities. These terms have never been stable, they shift constantly over time, and they may be just as uncertain and "social" as sociolegal descriptions of crime.[50] Moreover, how many behavioral incidents are required to establish a repetitive pattern of behavior? While ASPD criteria use terms like "inflexible" and "maladaptive," it is reasonable to ask if and how researchers apply these inexact descriptors to diagnose unique personal disorders, or to discern what really counts as a recurring or repetitive pattern of behavior. The neuroscientists I spoke with, however, are keenly attuned to this problem. Dr. Smith told me:

> A really big ongoing change in psychiatry and clinical psychology is to see clinical disorders, like for example conduct disorder, as continuous variable, not a category. Conduct problems vary. So, these things vary continuously in the population, and there aren't—as much as we would like there to be—discrete categories. We have to think of them as continuously distributed. Also, the current diagnostic categories in the DSM are not very scientific, and in fact, you could get two kids with the same diagnosis who have, in fact, totally different brain processes going on. Or two kids with different diagnoses who, in fact, if you look at what's going on at a neural level, are very similar. And so, we need to back up from these diagnostic categories and realize that they're not—they're not the gold standard.[51]

Thus, researchers may look to the *DSM* to help establish diagnostic criteria as a way to avoid the seemingly exclusive or exceptional forms of violence, but neither the production nor the employment of these biomedical classifications resolves the tension inherent in the schema.

MEASURABILITY: THE QUANTIFICATION OF VIOLENCE

Identifying patterns is just one step. Fitting also requires *measurability*, which necessitates the development of quantified values of violence. Neuroscientists read patterns of violence as symptoms through a complex observation methodology that involves neuropsychological scales to sort through, compute, and assign appropriate values of behavior. Neuropsychological scales help to quantify and standardize the subjective practices of diagnosis to be more accurate, objective, and reliable. To exemplify the importance of quantifying violence, I will focus on Robert Hare's Psychopathy Checklist (PCL-R), one of the most frequently utilized and thoroughly tested psychological scales in the world.

Although psychopathy has never been an official *DSM* diagnosis, there are undeniable overlaps between it and the *DSM*'s antisocial personality disorder (ASPD). Both emphasize the risk for antisocial behavior, but psychopathy explains this behavior as an effect of emotional deficits, such as lack of empathy.[52] Yet the ambiguities, both between and within the respective categories, have been a major point of contention and critique concerning the use of them as diagnoses.[53] Recent guidelines for ASPD in the United Kingdom continue to circumvent imperative questions about the ontological uncertainty of the classification, which risk reifying ASPD as a stable and unproblematic diagnostic category and increase the possibility of both overdiagnosis and misdiagnosis of the category in vulnerable populations like at-risk youth.[54] Pickersgill notes that the closeness and distance between the categories change over time as a result of "path dependency"—"the means by which decision-making in innovation is shaped by earlier choices, even when these lack salience in new settings."[55] He demonstrates this point through an excavation of memos and official organization minutes from the American Psychiatric Association (APA) on the use of antisocial personality disorder in its official manual, the *DSM*.[56] In doing so, he makes clear that the ontological challenges make complete stabilization of these diagnostic meanings of violence an impossible task.

Psychopathy is detected through the use of the PCL-R and other similar psychological scales. In a sense, this disorder symbolizes one's psychological

score. The PCL-R is a twenty-point interview-based tool that quantifies behavioral traits. Each item on the checklist can be scored on a three-point
scale (0 = clearly not present; 1 = maybe present; 2 = clearly present), and
psychopathy scores range from 0 to 40.[57] Although the PCL-R yields a numerical value for psychopathy, the actual determination of the classification
is not so straightforward. An assessment of PCL-R scores is obtained from
semi-structured interviews between patient and psychologists in combination with an examination of the patient's/offender's institutional record.
The behavioral records help to demonstrate whether particularly patterns of
behavior are present, and the interview enables researchers to determine the
proper weight (0, 1, or 2) for each of the PCL-R questions.

Psychopathy scores are not only values, but contentious zones of knowing
the signs of a lack of empathy, remorse, or conscience. Psychopathy cutoff
scores for neuroimaging violence studies that I analyzed varied. There is
no consensus about what numerical value is the "right" cutoff point. Some
studies used a score of 23 or 25 as the cutoff; individuals with scores at or
above these levels were designated as psychopathic, and individuals below
them were enrolled as the study's control group. Others used more cautious
cutoffs for psychopathy, a PCL-R score of 30 or above for psychopathy and a
score of 20 or below for the control population.[58] Such precautions help prevent misclassification and ensure a cleaner distinction between psychopathic
and non-psychopathic (normal) groups, and a more informative analysis for
neuroimaging studies. Still, inconsistencies in the use of psychopathy cutoff
scores prevent proper comparisons across neuroimaging studies.[59] Part of
this speaks to the cultural sensitivities that affect the use of the psychopathy checklist outlined above. Recent studies on inter-rater reliability on the
PCL-R reveal that scores are not always consistent across researchers, and
that scoring variability is dependent upon the interviewer's gender, country
of origin, training, and education.[60] The critique of PCL-R here is not aimed
at its utility in assessing psychopathy properly, but instead asks, *What does
it mean for the PCL-R to work?*

Quantitative interpretations of behavioral and pre-behavioral traits are
thought to better capture scientific reason, validity, and objectivity; thus
quantified factors of the studied phenomena are rendered the only factors
important for the study. As Theodore Porter notes, "Strategies of quantification work in an economy of personal and public knowledge, of trust and

suspicion."[61] Here, then, the goal of fitting is not to distinguish *the* value of psychopathy; instead fitting involves developing a range of values between psychopathy and the normal—"an optimal middle within a spectrum of variation."[62] In this way, each lab can employ its own "work-around"—a "local solution to the problems posed by global standardization."[63] In the case of the PCL-R, local work-arounds are demonstrated by the often arbitrary numerical cutoff values that allow each lab to piece together its own neurobiological interpretation of psychopathy. Thus, researchers do not have to prove why a 30 is a 30, why a 29 is a radically different "kind" than a 30, or why a 20 is seemingly more normal than a 25, but only that a score of 30 "fits" both the psychological criteria for and the social expectation of a psychopath.[64] This is not to imply that neuroscientists have not found links between the brain and the assemblage practices and dispositions known as psychopathy, but it does make it harder to compare and corroborate the findings across the literature. In essence, work-arounds help impose a sense of clarity in the shorthand without fully dealing with the inherent messiness and uncertainties that beset psychopathy scales.

QUALIFIERS: PUTTING WORDS TO THE NUMBERS

Qualifying adjectives for aggression can also be used to better achieve fit. The goal of this move is to simplify which kinds of persistent offenders matter and to demonstrate that unique neurobiological factors can be linked to specific personality disorders. Researchers see a correlation between the concepts of aggression and violence. In this aspect of the fitting process, specific types of aggression first reinforce the philosophy that criminality naturally exists. Second, these qualities are used to help decipher how material differences between groups—like populations of people characterized as having ASPD or psychopathy—matter. They put words to the numbers, which then can help researchers better find fit.

Neurobiological research examines two distinct sub-types of aggression: impulsive and instrumental.[65] Dr. Garrett described the differences between the two in our interview as follows:

> Reactive [or impulsive] aggression is sort of emotionally aroused aggression, aggression in response to a perceived threat, or to frustration at the absence of a reward. It's hot-headed, emotionally-aroused, whereas the

proactive or instrumental aggression is more cold-blooded, using aggression to get what that person wants in a planned, instrumental fashion, whether that's sex or money or whatever. They use aggression in a planned way to get that desired outcome.

Moreover, both impulsive aggression and instrumental aggression have been linked to specific populations. As explained here by Dr. Fitzpatrick,

> instrumental aggression is if you use violence as a means to an end, that is, outside the violent act. I want your money, so I hit you to get your wallet, but I'm not interested primarily in hitting you. I just want your wallet. If you just give it to me, I'll be happy with that. That's typical of criminals, especially psychopaths.

Psychopathic individuals are thought to be especially susceptible to demonstrating this goal-directed type of aggression due to impairments in the affect system, especially in relation to moral thoughts and behaviors. Psychopathic traits, including instrumental aggression, have been linked to areas of the brain that control emotions, most commonly the brain's amygdala region.[66] However, even with the addition of these two characteristics for aggression, there are still difficulties pertaining to their use, and their associations with *DSM* disorders are not straightforward.

This is especially apparent when psychopaths are understood to exhibit *both* instrumental and impulsive forms of aggression, as is widely believed now. Additionally, discrepancies in such classifications can be captured through technologies, which researchers must then decide how best to interpret. Here again, Dr. Garrett's explanation helps us contextualize this point:

> There's a distinction between impulsive violence, which is found in a lot of disorders, and instrumental violence, which is kind of typical of psychopathy and its predecessors in childhood so-called "callous and unemotional traits"—or kids who torture animals, and that kind of stuff. That's different, I think, and also different in terms of brain mechanisms behind it, so I believe it is a meaningful distinction. It was actually an interesting discovery, because when the genetic association between monoamine oxidase A (MAOA) and violence was observed in the epidemiological studies, this interpretation leaned toward instrumental violence, criminality. But what we saw in the brain very clearly showed that what

carriers of this variant had was a pattern of brain activation that was only consistent with a disposition towards *impulsive* violence, you know? So, they had hyperactivation of emotional brain regions, decreased regulation of those emotional brain regions by prefrontal areas—all things that you see in people who are impulsive. And they were, in fact, impulsive. So that made a lot more sense this way around.

Dr. Garrett helps us understand how the brain operates as a technology in the fitting process, an optimal site to interpret the true biosocial meaning of violence. The associations made between these forms of aggression and specific disorders are continually being remade, further clarified through discoveries in neurobiology, which researchers can use to help substantiate earlier diagnoses. Thus, the practices undergirdingg the fitting process do not have to be precise, as it is expected that these understandings will be further refined over time, through neurotechnologies and practices.

Qualifying behavioral characteristics are also used to formulate specific subpopulations for study. These divisions go beyond *DSM* classifications, and are used in experimental practices to further refine biomedical traits of violence. In one study, neuroscientists divided psychopaths into two groups on the basis of criminal convictions: "unsuccessful" psychopaths (individuals who were prosecuted for crimes) and "successful" psychopaths (individuals who had avoided any legal convictions—i.e., they were not caught). After scanning, the researchers found significant difference in the amygdala and prefrontal cortex regions of "unsuccessful" psychopaths compared to those of "successful" psychopaths and normal control groups. While the authors note that the qualifiers "successful" and "unsuccessful" refer only to criminal convictions, the study elucidates the continued salience of criminal justice or legal terminology in the neurobiology of violence. Criminal convictions may help neuroscientists detect a pattern of behavior, but these data alone do not capture all violent or criminal acts; some violent acts may go unreported and undetected, while others may reflect abusive or discriminatory patterns of law enforcement. It also important to note here that the use of criminal convictions is prevalent in this research, even though the stated goal is to move away from a sociolegal framework toward more-clinical, and seemingly more-objective, measures of behavior. What we find, and will see again later, is that biology does not supersede the sociological or cultural ways of knowing the criminal; instead, such ideas insidiously work their way into this neurobiological schema of violence.

What we are observing is the complex synthesis of biological, sociocultural, and clinical standards. While researchers strive to limit neurobiological research to measurable phenotypes, which are seemingly more realizable and biologically real than criminal justice labels, we see that the use of "abstract" legal and social qualifiers like "unsuccessful" or "successful" strategically work their way back into the fitting process. Thus the same subjective bias that researchers are trying to reduce comes into their favor here when they need to pull back on such dynamics in order to "fit."

This also causes us to revisit Duster's ontological critique, that the program takes for granted the socially contingent definition of violent behavior. However, Duster's cogent assessment is not simply telling us that violence is a social category; it is instead reminding us that it is a sociopolitical one. Memorialized within the categorization of violence is a contested history, an expressly gendered and racialized politic that often reinforces normatively hierarchical social arrangements based upon these powerful social practices. Thus the program's inability to deal with sociocultural contingencies, or with the persistent definitional ambiguities inherent in the classifications of violence, denies the category of "violence" or "aggression" or "anti-sociality" from operating in either natural or neutral terms. For Duster, the closest resemblance of a warrant for the research program relies less on any true theoretical justification and more on a teleological one that arises from a sense of empiricism. The mere existence of a prior biology of violence, and biological factors of violence, has been enough to authorize the warrant for continued study of such behaviors with advanced scientific practices.

Here I am trying to dig into this question a bit more. The social practices of this science tied to recruitment, classifications, measurability, violence attributes, or qualifiers help to show that researchers are not just relying on prior biology of violence but are remaking these ontological positions into a new ideal understanding of behavior. While these processes of fitting seem to generate stand-alone or objective boundaries of scientific exploration, they are actually bringing together older sociocultural understandings of violence and providing new scientific ways to realize, demarcate, and measure these traits and behaviors. Thus, the process of fitting sinks into the infrastructure of the research, always operating in the background through the (re)articulation of subjects, the (re)mapping of epistemic boundaries, and the (re)gauging of technological tools.

Interestingly, the attempt to better contextualize, or rationalize, the study of violence, also poses several empirical uncertainties that need to be managed and negotiated for the next step. Therefore, practices of fitting help to create and bolster assurance that behaviors, people, and brains in which scientists are interested have viable neurobiological import. Fitting, then, is never really complete. Instead, it continues to reinforce neuroscientists' confidence in the making of the "violent brain."

3 "PICTURING" RISKY BRAINS

IN THE EARLY SUMMER OF 1982, John Hinckley, Jr., was on trial for the attempted assassination of U.S. president Ronald Reagan. Hinckley's eventual acquittal prompted a national backlash and political calls for limitations on the insanity defense.[1] However, this case was also meaningful in another sense. Hinckley's attorneys requested that a computed tomography (CT) scan be admitted into evidence as proof of his schizophrenia diagnosis. This marked the first time that brain scans would be used as evidence in a U.S. criminal trial.[2] However, it was not without controversy.

The prosecution rejected the idea, arguing that CT scans as a diagnostic tool lacked consensus acceptance from the scientific community and therefore should not be admitted into evidence. Initially, it seemed as if federal district judge Barrington Parker, who presided over the trial, supported the prosecution's objection. Judge Parker admonished the defense's key witness, Harvard psychiatrist David Bear, when Bear refused to continue his testimony without reference to the CT images taken of Hinckley's brain. At one point, Judge Parker reportedly told Bear, "You are not in a classroom; you are in a courtroom . . . [and] bound by the rules of the court." Later, during a bench conference with the attorneys, Judge Parker again expressed displeasure with Bear's testimony, first threatening to hold him in contempt of court, then adding that Bear was not going to "twist things around . . . he is not up there lecturing with some intellectuals at Harvard."[3] Yet, just a few weeks later, Judge Parker softened his stance and allowed the CT scans into evidence, apparently noting that excluding the scans would "deprive the jury of the complete picture" of Hinckley's mental state.[4]

The use of Hinckley's CT scans in the courtroom acted as a powerful "expert image."[5] CT imaging employs a series of X-ray beams to produce images in much finer detail than standard X-ray technology alone. Defense experts drew upon this technological gain to make sense of their diagnosis of Hinckley's mental state. For example, neuroradiologist Marjorie LeMay testified that Hinckley's brain scan showed abnormally wide sulci—referring to the grooves or fissures on the surface of the human brain that gives it the distinct bumpy appearance. LeMay's statements helped corroborate Bear's prior testimony, which suggested that Hinckley's abnormal brain structure was an indication of the "organic brain disease" schizophrenia.[6] This information suggested that the experts were privy to hidden cerebral signs of abnormality via the technological assistance. Thus, the necessity for this evidence in the courtroom was framed as self-evident proof of Hinkley's mental state by researchers; yet—and paradoxically—the courtroom audience needed the interpretation, explanation from an actual human expert, in order to grasp its salience. And even then, it was unclear if and how these images affected the jury's decision to acquit in spite of other evidence in the case.

The use of visual technologies in the Hinckley trial deepened debates about the relationship between mental illness and crime instead of resolving them. Back-to-back headlines ran in the *New York Times* aptly capturing how these complex courtroom arguments were presented to the public. An article published June 2, 1982, "Cat Scans Said to Show Shrunken Hinckley Brain," appeared after Judge Parker allowed the scans into evidence. Just two days later, however, the newspaper seemingly reversed its prior headline after the prosecution's experts were called to rebut the neurobiological evidence from Bear's and LeMay's testimonies; "Hinckley's Brain Is Termed Normal," read the headline.[7] The point here illustrates the power of the visual, the necessity for expert readings of these images, and particularly how these new technologies brought together the notions of "seeing" and "knowing" in a simplistic yet effective way.

The introduction of Hinckley's brain scans at trial foreshadowed future and ongoing internal disputes within the psy-sciences about the brain, mental illness, and criminal culpability. It also highlighted concerns about the public consumption and scrutiny of such knowledges. Most important for our conversation, the use of neuroscientific evidence in the courtroom, especially the links drawn between the brain (size and shape) and mental disorders, is directly tied to the eventual emergence of neuroimaging research on violence.

Starting in the late 1980s, psychology slowly began to incorporate neuroimaging alongside, and sometimes in place of, traditional behavioral methods to validate the material basis of long-standing theories about the human psyche.[8] As cognitive neuroscientist Michael Gazzaniga states, "Human brain imaging suddenly appeared on the scene, and with it, the ability to study the human brain in action. Everything from basic issues in perception to higher order mental activities, were fair game for study."[9]

Throughout the 1990s, imaging technologies became a routine part of basic medical services, and MRI machines could be found in most major hospitals and university settings.[10] By 2000, however, proximity to these machines and improvements to open source data analysis spilled over to, and helped further energize, imaging for nonmedical practices, what neurologist Geoffrey Aguirre calls the "democratization of imaging."[11] This has meant that neuroimaging has been "readily adopted in new areas of intellectual inquiry without the need to bring along the hard-won cautionary experience that results from years of training and experience," according to Aguirre.[12] Likewise, neuropsychiatrist Ray Dolan adds that the democratization of imaging technologies fueled the exponential rise of neuroimaging research on questions of human cognition. "Most people would agree that democracy is a good thing," writes Dolan, "but equally, most people would agree that all things taken in excess should carry a health warning.[13] Such concerns should give us all pause when reading media reports purporting that neuroimaging allows political "campaigns to tap into the subconscious thoughts and feelings of potential voters."[14] They should force us to question discussions about the neural underpinnings of love when listening to our favorite podcasts, and think twice while perusing YouTube clips to learn how to "rewire" or "train" our brains for success.

In terms of the neuroimaging of violence, convenient access to scanner machines and data analysis software helps explain how this technology eventually emerged as the "right tool for the job."[15] However, the increased use of imaging in the psy-sciences is inseparable from funding. Modifications in scientific interests or practices shift according to changes in funders' priorities, institutional demands, and larger public policy concerns, not in a linear, casual manner.[16] A 2019 study examining funding proposals suggests that neuroscientists couch their research ideas in terms of "scientifically acknowledged conventions and paradigmatic requirements" to demonstrate their proficiency with regard to established scientific norms in the field.[17] Therefore, whether a project's focus is novel or aberrant may have less impact on grant decisions than the ability to convince grant reviewers that the project does not deviate from existing theories within the psy-sciences. With regard to the neuroimaging research on violent behaviors, there is evidence that such "loosely coupled and complex" relationships among researchers, funding agencies, academic institutions, and scientific innovation help to spur the upsurge of publications on the subject.[18]

From 1987 to 1999, there were fewer than 10 published peer-reviewed imaging studies on violence. In the same thirteen-year period, starting in 2000, however, the number of publications jumped to more than 90, and there were well over 180 new articles published between 2013 and 2019.[19] Nearly all of these studies had multiple streams of funding, often reflecting the multiple number of researchers who contributed to the publication. A significant number of the articles cite funding, partially or fully, from national government agencies, like the U.S. National Institutes of Health and the UK Medical Research Council. This speaks volumes about the way views about the program have shifted today. I do not intend to imply that state-funded agencies and scientific peers today indiscriminately accept the knowledge claims produced from the neuroscience of violence. However, compared to the program's past, the use of established neuroscientific (and genetic) techniques and adoption of similarly respected claims about the brain and cognition, have better helped rationalize, or legitimize, the biological study of violence.

VISUALIZATION AS "TOOL"

The power to visualize has always played a vital role for biological research on violence. Phrenology (ascertaining personality traits from the contours of the skull), craniometry (measurements of skull size), somatology (observations of bodily shape), and even photography (e.g., mug shots) are technologies used to construct an image of the violent subject. Inconsistencies and questionable findings have riddled each of these visual tools—a fact that contemporary researchers acknowledge when they denounce such technological setbacks as "pseudoscientific" or flawed endeavors that ultimately damaged the image of the biology of violence. Nevertheless, researchers still rely upon such technical assistance, as it is thought to facilitate a special style of scientific authority that permits researchers to inspect the body for the roots of deviancy with objective clarity.

New technologies hold the promise to help researchers move past the program's old flaws. However, flawed attempts of the past are not fully discarded, but are refashioned as "key historical period[s] when the *right* questions were being asked, with the *wrong* technologies."[20] With each stride along the path to "scientific progress," researchers believe they are better able to detect and uncover the root causes of violence, now supposedly tucked away in genetic code or neural circuitry. Critiques of past technologies, then, serve a pragmatic purpose. They act as reflection points to help demonstrate the progression of the science, and help preserve, in a reflexive manner, key ontological foundations that help to guide the development and focus of new technologies and practices. There is little doubt that the technologies of today are more sophisticated and widely accepted throughout science and medicine. That is, today's technologies are not simply yesteryear's phrenology. However, these new visual technologies are not necessarily discovering new objective facts about violence, either.

During Lombroso's era, the knowable signs of violence were believed to lie in common sense. Historian David Horn writes that "artists, writers, the 'lower class,' and even children, according to Lombroso, were aware of and could reproduce in painting and poems the contours of criminal physiognomy."[21] Lombroso's assertions, while absurd, can also be read as a tacit acknowledgment that he did recognize criminality (its meaning, not its etiology) as a product of sociocultural interactions. In contrast, today's researchers are less concerned with criminal character as a depiction of the outer flesh. This is due, at least in part, to the abilities of neuroimaging—the powerful visual technologies that have become commonplace in both scientific representations and public interpretations of the brain. Today's *neuro-criminologic gaze* promises to heighten the eye's prowess, enabling researchers to detect differences not just upon the flesh or under the skull, but seemingly those that are invisible to our normal senses.

Imaging technologies—MRI, fMRI, PET—have excelled as a result of their ability to "see" and replicate brain function and structure in iconic brain images. Scientific authority of these technologies, and brain scans, rests on the idea that researchers can literally visualize (neuro)biological signs of risk that are undetectable to laypeople. However, these technologies are not actually directly recording or capturing live "pictures" of brains. Neuroimaging is an ongoing, and sometimes iterative, relationship between social cooperation and technical dependency. Thus, it is a social practice.

The best way to understand this point is to put yourself in the shoes of a study participant. At the beginning of each interview I asked participants to provide an explanation of a normal imaging experiment. Below, I share Dr. Hollowell's succinct description of "what happens in the scanner" during a functional MRI experiment seeking to understand how the brain processes particular emotions thought to be associated with aggressive and impulsive violent behaviors:

> The first thing you want to do is make sure that [participants] don't get freaked out by being in the scanner, because it's enclosed. So, we have a mock scanner. We make sure people are comfortable in there, because if you're really claustrophobic, you can't be scanned, and we can't study you. That's one day. On another day, [participants] will come in, and we [will] put them in the [actual] MRI scanner. They're going to be looking at a screen with those fancy glasses that allow them to lie in the machine without sitting up. And they'll have some earphones because there may be some instructions or sounds. Then the machine will start doing its thing while they're just sitting there to get a baseline scan. Then when the task starts, participants will typically—if it's an emotion-information processing task, which often happens—see a bunch of faces of a certain emotion. The participant may even be asked to state what kind of emotion they saw—was it a positive emotion or a negative emotion. Then there'll be a rest period. After, they'll be shown a different group of pictures. At the end of the study, we will look at the activation when they were looking at certain kinds of pictures. The angry pictures versus happy faces or sad faces. And that's pretty much what happens in the scanner.[22]

There is more to this practice, as explored below. Nevertheless, this short description does provide a glimpse of the relationship between participants and researchers. Study participants are not necessarily passive bodies, leisurely resting under the magnet while they await their "picture" to be taken. During this process they are expected to be "docile patients," and their bodies are disciplined to be more receptive to medical procedures.[23] Imaging participants must be willing to follow directions: remaining still throughout the scan, listening to the technician's directions, responding to the task correctly. Participants who cannot adhere to these rules, those who cannot remain motionless during the scan, or those who are described as claustrophobic or just noncompliant, are often omitted from studies, since essentially their brain scans cannot be trusted during this stage of the science. Therefore, trust is a vital step in realizing the neurobiological correlates of violence. Trust that a participant's brain is acceptable for scanning correctly, trust that technologies will operate properly, and, as we will see, trust that scientists themselves can interpret neuronal activity accurately.

Researchers who use imaging to study violence are tasked with navigating the practical constraints of these machines, while also trying to prove that such data provide the best chance to understand the causes of violence. This raises an important question: If, and how, can neuroscientists balance the immense benefits of scanning technologies and products, on the one hand, from the potential technical and epistemological limits of these compelling research materials, on the other? A likely answer to this question lies in the way neuroscientists contextualize the role of imaging in relation to other modes of research in the field. For example, neuroscientist Dr. Holmes cautioned during our interview that neuroimaging is "just *one tool in the toolbox* of neuroscience, and still quite a young and crude tool, so I wouldn't put too much emphasis on that."[24] He issued this warning when I asked about the way neuroscientists make sense of differences picked up in the scanner—although it is not clear why he decided to provide this description at this particular time, given that I had asked other questions about imaging practices earlier in the interview. Conceivably, his response served as a general pushback against myopic views of the neurosciences that perceive neuroimaging as the epitome of the field as a whole—which Dr. Holmes may have regarded as my view as well. Other researchers I talked with also noted the technical limits of explaining violence through scientific visualizations, and especially the likely misuses and misunderstandings in the public sphere. Therefore, in this limited sense, Dr. Holmes's toolbox analogy is appropriate, as it helps to demonstrate and contextualize researchers' recognition of the limits of this "crude tool." At the same time, however, neuroscientists in this program also trust in, and sometimes rely too much on, the power of visualization to justify their work.

The turn to imaging has helped to improve funding opportunities for biological research on violence from national-level governmental agencies. Additionally, the use of neuroimaging has been beneficial for researchers themselves, especially those who have gained prestige in the field of neuro-psychology and in society in general through new roles as public intellectuals and important expert witnesses in high-profile criminal cases. The remaining question, however, is this: what do visual representations of data add, if any-thing, to the dissemination of knowledge about a constantly shifting, ever political set of behaviors like violence? Visual representations of biological data may more effectively communicate a sense of objectivity and fact-ness, beyond other forms of data presentation. In this more comprehensive sense, then, brain imaging is by no means an ordinary gadget in the neuroscience "toolbox."

In order to fully appreciate the importance of this argument, we must also attend to the larger ethics concerns of imaging. Specifically, let us turn to the broader conversation about the public's interpretation of biological information. There is evidence from research studies that the inclusion of neuroscientific data, even irrelevant data, to an explanation can increase the chance that an individual will perceive that explanation as more logical and believable.[25] Conversely, a recent study has found that the addition of biological data about psychopathy did not affect sentencing decisions made by a mock jury.[26] The most appropriate interpretation of the public's take on biological knowledge probably lies somewhere in between these two findings.

It is probable that public audiences are more likely to accept a neurosci-entific explanation "when it confirms prior beliefs."[27] Social science research on genetics and racial identity suggests that genetic ancestry information is regarded unevenly and subjectively by public audiences; thus, biological knowledges do not necessarily dictate or replace the public's own conceptions about identity or kinship.[28] While there is no predetermined manner in which the public will consider brain arguments about violent behavior, brain images convey, quite convincingly, epistemic validation. Their presentation to the research field and to the public is much different from the way genealogical DNA maps are presented in statistical tables and charts.

These visualizations help to manage complexity, both in the lab and in public settings, and also help develop greater scientific and empirical capital in the biology of violence. Brain scans serve as an interface to connect, and make meaning between, the bodies placed under a scanner and the intricate computational output of the scanner. They "are not images or pictures to be passively looked at, but material to be experimented with."[29] As research materials, brain scans act as strategic points of coordination, engagement, and interaction. During the production of the science, scans help re-assemble and fine-tune practices of fitting to provide a particular model of violence. Once disseminated, both within and beyond the bounds of the program, these images help to simplify the purported biological foundations of violent behaviors.[30]

The aesthetic attraction of brain scans, therefore, can be misleading, as it "invite[s] us to believe" in an epistemic power that is often beyond the functional limit of the technology.[31] Moreover, our acceptance of this "invitation" to visually know ourselves is often routine and even anticipated. Thus, it is likely that imaging can more effectively communicate the epistemic value of neuroscience research—that brains actually do "light up," scans really are "pictures" of brains, and, importantly, neuroscientists actually can noninvasively "see" and make sense of living brains with remarkable precision. Scans cultivate a greater conviction for "seeing" humanness—bodies, minds, identities, and experiences—as a primary product of the neural senses, fostering a "multiplication of witnesses" to the powers of the brain.[32] The incorporation of imaging practices helped to reshape the program in a much more productive light than in the past, and ostensibly helped to legitimate the research as essential for progress in health, science, and justice. Thus, neuroimaging has extended the authority of the *gaze* like never before.

Foucault captured this dynamic in modern medicine, using the term "medical gaze," and his critique has been aptly applied to criminology as well.[33] For him, the gaze represented a shift in medicine, in which this body is transformed into a site of knowing. The gaze operates in a seemingly self-evident fashion, as it anchors the making, and validation, of logical certainty in clinical and research practices. Moreover, Foucault's gaze infers a mode of disciplining, a discursive technique of power that produces particular types of bodies.[34] Delineating a Foucauldian critique of medicalization, sociologist Deborah Lupton states: "The central strategies of disciplinary power are observation, examination, measurement, and the comparison of individuals against an established norm, *bringing them into a field of visibility*."[35] The gaze simultaneously reconstitutes and rationalizes the abilities of the "knower" (doctor/neuropsychologist) to detect (see), and through a homogenizing discourse it reduces the "object" (patient/criminal) to knowable signs, markers, measures to be seen or discovered.[36] Thus, the clinician's ability to observe the hidden or imperceptible sources of illness represents a specific kind of belief system enacted through a complex set of power relations between doctor and patient, neuropsychologist and (would-be) criminal. However, neither the gaze nor visual technologies alone are sufficient to decipher the salience of the neuroscience of violence. As science and technology studies (STS) scholar Michael Lynch notes, "visualization is as much the work of hands—often many hands—as it is the so-called gaze."[37]

In a coordinated and flexible manner, the neurocriminologic gaze, imaging technologies, and the fitting process all together help to produce the authoritative construct that I call the *violent brain* model. The violent brain is less a material substrate than it is an "ideal type"—that is, this construct is supposedly reflective of the known biological characteristics of a violent person, and yet also equipped to project, or "discover" in scientific terms, the potential neurobiological determinants of violence and the expected scientific and social uses for these knowledges. The realization, manipulation, and expectation of this construct presents a malleable, and arguably more convincing, biological platform for tracing the etiology of violent behaviors. Neuroscientific understanding and expectation of what a "violent" person's brain is or should be are made in formation of this ideal, such that "facts" about violence, the brain, and risk are accepted a priori of the experimental procedures, then enacted, realized, through the process of research and presentation of results. Moreover, in the process of formulating and enacting this model of violence, neuroscientists also seem to reenvision the material brain—the inaccessible raw material that researchers ostensibly experimented with or upon invasively through using imaging technologies. Through the violent brain model, researchers envision the material brain as the primary source of intervention and speculation—both the question and the solution for violence, the place to unearth facts about violence, and as shown in later chapters, the site at which to predict and potentially cure violence as well. Both this argument about the material brain and the larger role of this new construct, the violent brain, become more clear through a review of the way the neuroscientific study of violence has evolved alongside technological advances in imaging.

THE BRAINS OF "MURDERERS"

By the end of the 1980s newer imaging approaches, like positron emission tomography (PET), had started to replace CT technologies, which were used in the Hinckley trial, and expanded the psy-sciences' interests in the brains of violent subjects. Unlike CT scans, which focus on brain structure, PET imaging uses radioactive tracers to indirectly ascertain brain function. During the scan, the machine detects gamma rays emitted from these tracers as an indication of metabolic activity, a sign that the observed brain area is "active."

A key asset of this model of violence is the ability to visually show differences. To be fair, we must admit that neurobiological logics of violence are less interested in distinguishing the "good" from the "bad," although traces of this ontology are forever instilled in the practices of this research program. The violent brain model, instead, seeks to visualize the "seeds of violence" within the good, the bad, and populations in-between.[38] This was a point that came up during my interview with Dr. Moore, whom I asked to reflect on some things that were well understood about the use of neuroimaging to study violence, and on issues that still need to be addressed. After commenting on the increased utility of MRIs, resulting from lower costs and advancements in computer software, Dr. Moore outlined the diagnostic dilemma with imaging:

> In terms of the biological differences, what to do if you find them. That is [the] tricky bit. How to diagnose the disorder—you can diagnose the disorder clinically, but I don't think we're at the level where you can do an MRI scan and suggest that you're picking up differences in this brain region, and that this corresponds to a psychopath. I don't think we're there yet. And I'm not sure we ever will be there, because that involves investigating a lot of people over a long period of time and coming up with consistent areas of abnormality. And I think we're still very much in the early days of that frontier in research.[39]

Dr. Moore's argument makes clear that imaging, at this time, is an unreliable diagnostic tool. The "tricky bit" outlined here can also be discussed in terms of "reverse inference." Reverse inference "reasons backwards from the presence of brain activation to the engagement of a particular cognitive function."[40]

Neuroscientist Russell Poldrack compares reverse inference to a person having a fever. He notes that the presence of a fever is often regarded as a reliable sign of disease or infection. However, since a fever is a recognized symptom for myriad diseases and conditions, its mere presence cannot identify the specific disease or infection that is afflicting the patient; it can only indicate that the individual may be ill.[41] Similarly, for reverse inference to be most useful, the cognitive process in question must be unique—the only cause for activation—to the specified brain region.[42] Therefore, activation in a particular brain region for, say, a group of violent individuals, and not the control group, only demonstrates differences in activation. This also suggests that the particular area is related to some cognitive trait ostensibly associated with the violent individual group, but researchers cannot conclude definitively that the region is the cause of violence.

One of the earliest imaging studies on violence examined brain function in a group of people characterized by both mental illness and a history of violent behavior.[43] Although this study's sample included only four patients, all of whom were diagnosed with concomitant psychiatric disorders and/or habitual drug or alcohol abuse, psychologists Nora Volkow and Laurence Tancredi's study opened an intriguing line of inquiry that became vital for future neuroimaging studies of violence. It suggested that structurally "healthy" brains may require further inspection in order to see the expected causal factors for violence. Two of the patients in the study had relatively normal CTs, but PET scans indicated greater functional deficits in their frontal lobes compared with those of the other two patients in the study, both of whom had abnormal CT results.[44] Thus, Volkow and Tancredi demonstrated that PET scans could help detect irregularities that went unnoticed with structural brain scans like CT.

This vision of the brain's hidden potentials, or in this case irregularities, intensified in the 1990s as PET was more regularly adopted as the method used to visualize the brains of violent offenders. Adrian Raine—then a professor of psychology at the University of Southern California—and colleagues published a series of PET studies on murderers from 1994 to 1998.[45] In contrast to the mental health populations used in studies like Volkow and Tancredi's, Raine's team shifted their attention, ever so slightly, to individuals who were defined *first* by their criminal behavior (e.g., murderers) and *second* by their mental ill-health. Their participants were (mostly) men who had been referred by the court for psychological evaluation. All participants had either pled not guilty by reason of insanity (NGRI) for murder or manslaughter or had already been convicted of murder or manslaughter and were awaiting psychological evaluation for sentencing purposes.

The series of imaging studies conducted by Raine and colleagues highlighted the reliance on psychological tasks for functional imaging. Neuropsychological tasks help researchers evaluate a participant's cognitive abilities and, when paired with brain imaging, are thought to help researchers recognize better unique responses from specified areas of the brain.[46] Raine's group used the continuous performance task (CPT), which assesses impulsivity and attention. Poor performance on the CPT can suggest compromised executive functioning, which tells neuroscientists that an individual may have abnormalities in the prefrontal and temporal brain lobes.[47] Murderers in this study did show reduced brain activity in the prefrontal cortex (PFC)—a brain region linked to several higher-order processes such as memory, decision making, and learning—which may indicate an increased susceptibility to violent behavior.[48] However, the research team found no differences between their study and normal groups on CPT; nevertheless, the task played a role in interpreting the findings.[49] Raine and colleagues wrote:

> The fact that groups did not differ in behavioral performance on the CPT suggests not only that difference in brain functioning is not easily accounted for by motivational or attentional deficits in the murderers, but also that the significantly greater occipital activity [the area associated with vision] in murderers may possibly represent compensation for the reduced activity in the prefrontal cortex.[50]

This is an example of the management of scientific uncertainty as rationalized through the image of the violent brain, which often complicates logic that equates technological advancements with greater empirical clarity. Scientific explanations are always contingent, on forces, decisions, and discourses that go beyond what may be viewed as official scientific experimentation.[51] Neuroscientists emphasize, reject, or seek alternate rationales for differences that they find because of prior knowledge—theoretical, empirical, and cultural—about the individual(s) in question, which is also interdependent with the way "violent" or "normal/healthy" groups are made and defined during the fitting process. Classifications, as we saw in Chapter 2, act as a type of pre-imaging framework to understand the expected actions, emotions, and tendencies thought to characterize violence. However, such rubrics can also distract us from questioning the assertions made during and after scanning that help researchers read differences into brains.[52]

Even though there were no demonstrated differences on the CPT between the control and target groups, Raine's team drew upon its function to attribute the success of "murderers" on the CPT task to brain regions, the occipital lobe, that were not directly measured in the study. The apparent lack of clarity in the experiment confirmed previously unseen, and unmeasured, brain qualities for the group of violent offenders. This explanation seems to suggest that PET imaging grasped a hidden understanding of violence that was not available with a task or behavioral method alone. Such deliberations, however, are not necessarily uncharacteristic or inappropriate to imaging.

Several contingent elements must be taken into consideration when trying to interpret the meanings of brain scans. Dr. Garrett's discussion of the ecological validity problem in our interview helps to clarify this point:

> You can argue the view that there is an ecological validity problem. You know, there are other things to take into account. Functional imaging scans have looked at the way [study groups] struggle to be conditioned by punishment information. The difficulty is that we know that these individuals are bad at behavior conditioned by punishment, so the change you see in the brain scans could just be that they're doing the task really badly. In the task that we use, we know that the behavior isn't responding as well as normal and that's without a [mental health diagnosis]. So, any brain changes that we see can't be related to just that change in behavioral difference.[53]

Ecological validity refers to how well the scientific findings can be generalized to the larger public, or a specific sphere of the public. Beyond generalizability, however, there remains a question about the way researchers reach empirical certainty when making and interpreting brain data.

What often becomes significant about the violent brain is bound to what is assumed to be known about such brains in the first place. Knowledge about "bad conditioning" led Dr. Garrett's lab to question the differences found in brain scan results, and the lack of differences in the CPT steered Raine and colleagues toward differences in another area of the brain. Raine, who reported that his own PET scan resembles certain traits of the murderers' brains in his study, certainly understands the delicate parsing of meanings required to understand images of brains.[54] He, like the other scientists I spoke with, often reiterate that neuroscientific studies do not rule out other (i.e., social) factors that are vital for understanding violence. If Raine's group considered that sociocultural dynamics may have influenced the CPT results, they did not indicate so in the article. Maybe, as Dr. Garrett mentions, they were trying to attenuate the possible effects of their participants' poor performance on the task. Yet such an adjustment and explanation do not explain why they privileged an unmeasured region of the brain.

SIZE (STILL) MATTERS

The Hinckley trial described above hinted at the role that brain size plays in attempts to link biology and violence. Scientific interest in the relationship between brain size and social traits dates back to at least the nineteenth century. Take, for example, the work of physician Samuel Morton, who amassed a collection of nearly a thousand human skulls to investigate differences in cranial capacity, his proxy for brain size. Racist preconceptions concerning the supposed biological differences in intelligence among racial groups tainted Morton's interest in brain capacity—as pointed out nearly a century later by evolutionary biologist Stephen J. Gould, who called Morton's *Craina Americana* project both racially biased and scientifically flawed.[55] Researchers at the University of Pennsylvania, where Morton's collection is preserved, recently retested Morton's measurements, and contrary to Gould's critique, they contend that Morton's methodology was neither biased nor flawed. [56] Morton, they argue, provides an example of how "the scientific method can shield results from cultural biases."[57] However, affirming Morton's measurements does not invalidate Gould's key argument. Morton's calculations can prove correct and so too can Gould's claim that Morton's *a priori* biases about "superior" and "inferior" racial groups dictated how he interpreted these findings.[58] Moreover, the fact that there remains controversy surrounding Morton's legacy serves as a reminder of the long and unwavering interest in understanding human health, behavior, and sociality through measurements of the brain.

Today's biology of violence also depends on the ability to link brain morphology (i.e., structure, shape, and volume) and social behavior. My point here is not to equate contemporary imaging research on violence to Morton's research practices or racist beliefs. Rather, I want to point out that the interpretation of this science also relies on a related heuristic of brain size. Around 2000, a new technology, magnetic resonance imaging (MRI), began to replace other forms of structural imaging (e.g., CT scans) in medical and research practices. MRI uses powerful magnetic fields to assess brain structure (sMRI) and it can be adapted to capture function (fMRI) as well. This technique provides greater spatial and temporal resolution than CT or PET, and the lack of radiation makes it a safer option than either of those techniques.[59] Like the above examples on PET imaging, however, neuroscientific interpretation of these values is neither neutral nor straightforward.

Let's turn again to Raine and colleagues, who provided one of the earliest structural magnetic resonance imaging procedures on antisocial behavior.[60] They examined percentage differences in volume of gray matter between groups diagnosed with antisocial personality disorder (ASPD) and three demographically different control groups.[61] Gray matter consists of the outer parts of the brain—the areas that contain neuron cell bodies, thought to be responsible for higher-level processes such as consciousness, memory, and decision making. Gray matter, therefore, is considered the area of the brain that is more closely associated with what makes us human. Neuroscientists studying violence through sMRI scans are interested in gray matter integrity (volume and structure) of regions thought to help manage our behavior. The link between gray matter and violent behavior rests on the logic that reduced gray matter volume or structurally abnormal gray matter may inhibit healthy or normal functioning of the region, which in turn limits the brain's ability to control unwanted behavior.

Raine's group found that the brains of men with ASPD had a lower percentage of gray matter than did those of the control groups. Thus their results confirm the hypothesized correlation between violent behavior and smaller brain volume. A close reading of the article also reveals the rationale used to make sense of these perceived differences in brain volume. They wrote:

> To our knowledge, this study establishes for the first time the existence of a subtle structural deficit in the prefrontal cortex of un-institutionalized antisocial, violent persons with psychopathic-like behavior. . . . It also

extends previous neurological research . . . by showing that a much less observable volume reduction specific to prefrontal gray matter is associated with [ASPD]. . . . [W]hile these effect sizes are thought to be large, *this deficit is visually imperceptible at a clinical radiological level.*[62]

These findings support Volkow and Tancredi's conclusions; here, brains may appear structurally "healthy" but have damage that can be picked up only through imaging. The key question about the presumed link between "smaller" brains and susceptibility to violence concerns *how much* of a reduction in gray matter must have occurred to deem brain malfunction a risk factor for violence.

In order to address this question, let us first consider the impact of Phineas Gage, a nineteenth-century American railroad worker who reportedly changed personality-wise due to a gruesome head injury that sent a tamping rod through the left side of his skull. Neuroimaging did not exist at the time, but researchers expect that the rod gouged out a substantial portion of the frontal part of his brain. The injury blinded Gage in the left eye and left a mark on his forehead, but remarkably he survived with little impairment to his memory, intelligence, or speech.[63] However, according to witnesses at the time, his personality was forever altered after the accident: Gage "was no longer Gage," they claimed, as the accident seemingly transformed him from a capable and well-respected railroad foreman into an ill-tempered and aggressive fellow.[64] And today Gage's brain continues to be the prototypical proof of the link between brain abnormality and behavior changes.

In 1994, a team of neuroscientists led by Hanna Damasio and Antonio Damasio analyzed Gage's preserved skull using neuroimaging technologies to help reconstruct the position of the tamping rod.[65] The group, working with what they posited as a digitized reconstruction of Gage's brain, observed a "neuroanatomical pattern" thought to have caused his behavioral changes. The part of the brain that they isolated, the ventral medial prefrontal cortex (vmPFC), is today correlated with abnormal decision making and behavioral changes. Other researchers have also relied on new interpretations of Gage's brain to support the neurobiological arguments about behavior.

Antonio Damasio, in his book *Descartes's Error*, refers to his patient "Eliot" as a "modern Phineas Gage."[66] Raine talks about the "Spanish Phineas Gage" in his book's chapter "Broken Brains."[67] And neuropsychiatrist Kent

Kiehl argues that Gage's condition was actually a precursor to modern-day psychopathy. Kiehl notes: "Neurologists originally named the condition [that] Gage suffered from *pseudopsychopathy*, but it was subsequently called *acquired sociopathic personality*. In other words, if you damage a part of the paralimbic system you can acquire a psychopathic personality."[68] The survival of Gage's story as proof of a specific brain-violence link, argues historian Peter Becker, "reduce[s] complex stories to a naked grid of references, which can easily circulate and be allied with other references to build new stories."[69] However, there is also another crucial point concerning the utility of Gage's retold narrative for neuroscience studies of violence: study participants do not have obvious brain lesions. In fact, the inclusion and exclusion criteria—i.e., the rules governing a study's recruitment of participants—for most neuroscientific research on violence expressly excludes participants with any known head injuries in the past to prevent any confounding effects. To rephrase the question from above, how much (or little) gray matter counts as "subtle differences" in the brain or the value of these minute differences compared to discernible lesions?

The use of MRI technologies became so vital to the program because they promised to detect *imperceptible* variances in brain structure. However, as Dr. Lewis explained to me in our discussion about the decision-making processes, the results of scans are delicate and quite malleable. In Dr. Lewis's words:

> What we understand is that the brain scanner can take pictures and help indicate how individuals who have a trait are different from individuals who don't have that trait. [Whether] the trait shows up as, you know, as a difference in the self-report scale, or differences in the neuropsychological test, or differences in the brain image, I think they're all about the same. The only question is if the brain image gives us a slightly more *intuitive kind of understanding* of where, when, and how, you know, [an individual] might have developed that abnormality.[70]

First, it is important to highlight Dr. Lewis's use of the term "pictures" to describe the highly complex, computer-produced visualizations—i.e., brain scans. Visualizing the neuropsychological dimensions thought to underpin the risk for violence as brain scans is not inherently deceptive. However, the routine use of terms like "pictures" increases the "attribution of false concreteness"—empirical certainty, regarding the meaning and function of the brain.[71] The presumption of "concreteness" paradoxically undermines the sociocultural value of this knowledge. Instead, place Dr. Lewis's use of the term "pictures" in context with the rest of the reply concerning the malleability afforded to researchers through these practices. The reference to "intuition" may be an attempt to convey the certainty of empiricism, but it actually exposes the ambiguity, as well as the continual need to produce and reaffirm scientific certainty.

Neuroscientific intuition, in this sense, means a combination of prior knowledges and training with presumably anticipated outcomes about abnormal brains and their impact on social behavior. An ongoing coordination among neuroscientists, research materials, and technologies is needed to produce and make sense of the violent brain prototype. This implicitly points to the fact that the production of neuroscientific accounts of violence is bound to, and indistinguishable from, the management of scientific uncertainty; thus, visualizing violence is a continual practice of negotiation that neither starts nor ends with brain scans. Therefore, this practice may also be reinterpreted as a product of the gaze. As Foucault reminds us, "To discover, therefore[,] will no longer be to *read* an essential coherence beneath a state of disorder, but to push a little farther back the foamy line of language . . . to introduce language into that penumbra where the gaze is bereft of words."[72]

The power of the gaze in the violent brain model, then, speaks directly to the way complex, and even antithetical, understandings of violence work through specific scientific practices to organize and structure what there is to see and interpret, and how such facts will and should matter. Thus, the seemingly unstructured nature of this empirical space is productive. What can be understood through the detection of the *imperceptible* or the neuroscientific reliance on "*an intuitive kind of understanding*" is that expected outcomes are often taken-for-granted assumptions that are situationally read into each tool through practice, which helps researchers to realize, in a seemingly rational and logical manner, the types of interpretive conclusions and solutions they should reach.

CAPTURING VIOLENCE "IN ACTION"

If the goal of sMRI is to generate an image of the structural foundations of violence in the brain, functional MRI (fMRI) attempts to provide the meaning of that picture. In fMRI, brain activity is captured as a measure of the ratio of oxygenated to deoxygenated blood, what is called a BOLD (blood-oxygen-level-dependent) signal. Shortly after a neuron fires, oxygen-rich blood is carried to these areas to replenish the energy depleted during brain activity. Oxygenated blood and deoxygenated blood react differently to magnetic fields, and the powerful magnets of the MRI can detect and measure these delicate changes to construct a representation of where activity is in the brain.[73] The more active the brain (or particular area of the brain), the more oxygen is required, and therefore the more blood flow.

Neuroscientists have been clear about the limits of this technology, but they still believe that fMRIs provide the best answers for violence right now. That is, fMRI is considered the most advanced technology in their "toolbox," but it is nevertheless still recognized that it is not necessarily a perfect tool. Take Dr. Smith's reply, for example, when I asked about the advantages and limitations of fMRI:

> So, with brain imaging we actually can see, you know, if two groups of different people seem to have different neural strategies to answer a common question. And, we can get some confirmation that's true. I mean—especially if you triangulate your data using lesion studies, animal studies and behavioral studies—you can draw pretty good conclusions about what the changes in blood flow mean. But you do have to be very careful because of course blood flow is not really the *brain in action*. Especially for more complicated questions. Are you measuring inhibitory neurons or excitatory neurons? Are you measuring what neurotransmitter systems are active in the regions you are looking at? Are there sub-populations of this big structure that are active? fMRI is better than anything else, but it's still not as good as it could be. *The fact is, blood flow is only a proxy for activation.*[74]

These comments make clear that the power of brain imaging does not rest on its ability to get everything accurate about the brain and violence, as "blood flow is only a proxy for understanding action." Neuroscientists have nevertheless turned to fMRIs, as they are "better than anything else," which I take to imply other neuroscientific tools. Articles citing the use of fMRI accounted for nearly half (47 percent) of all the articles I reviewed for my research. One reason why the use of fMRIs has increased the production of this science is that the ability to use blood flow to help illuminate the areas of the brain active during particular events or tasks has "revolutionized the kind of questions neuroscientists can ask" in relation to violent behavior.[75]

Enhancements to imaging are tightly bound to corresponding improvements to and the utility of neuropsychological tasks; thus imaging practices and their use of psychological tasks are coproduced. Take the "emotion-information processing" task described early in Dr. Hollowell's description of a typical imaging procedure. Researchers utilize different kinds of facial expressions to ensure that participants will infer the correct emotion and exhibit the proper neurobiological response during scanning. As Dr. Hollowell stated, "There's a happy face, sad face, or surprised face. And with the computer, we are able to make a neutral face, which is zero emotion, and a hundred-percent emotion face, like happy [face], and merge it so that you can have a variable face . . . it can go from being very, very sad to neutral to very happy or angry—whatever you want it to."[76] Activity detected in the brain when looking at computer-manufactured faces, like other tasks, is not a direct sign of violence, but an indicator that the brain area of interest is "active" during a specific emotive state. If it's an "angry" face, then any detected activity in the pre-selected brain area tells researchers something about the way this emotion is processed in the scanned individual. Most people can rationalize why scientists would consider emotions a precursor to violent behavior. However, the way neuroscientists approach the relationship between emotions and violence does not always reflect the rich and complex way they are expressed in social life.

Emotions that underlie social action can vary, and they are not easily parsed from social identities, environments, and engagements that help make and induce them in the first place. This is not to doubt the role that emotions play with regard to behavior, but to point out that these feelings or modes do not occur in isolation, and it would seem difficult to think about an emotion, like anger, in isolation when many other feelings and situations are needed to contextualize when it does, or does not, result in violent behavior. Reading emotions through the scanner—specifically the inducement, detection, and measurement of these affective states—guides researchers' decisions about what regions of the brain to focus on, or how to interpret the meanings of brain data. Also, there is a considerable body of literature on the neuroscience of emotions, so scientists are aware of these types of methodological hurdles and epistemological challenges.[77]

Researchers in the social and cognitive neurosciences do not claim to trace specific neuron activation to exact emotional states. Instead, this branch of neuroscience argues that fMRI, at best, can help researchers outline "neural reference spaces"—brain areas that are active during experiences of emotions.[78] Although this limitation is implicitly understood, its adherence can be lost or muddled in published articles. Here, the relationship between emotion and violent behavior reveals certain assumptions to which neuroscientists must subscribe in order to understand which responses should be valid, in this sense abnormal, for their study population. By linking emotions to specific areas of the brain, functional imaging articles can infer that researchers have identified the "real" culprit behind violent behavior: malfunctioning parts of the brain that fail to regulate behavior as they normally would. This complex interplay means that measures for violence, or the risk for violent behavior, are often assumed to be synonymous with impaired emotional regulation, an individual's "low threshold for activating negative affect (a mixture of emotions and moods that include anger, distress, and agitation) and a failure to respond appropriately to the anticipated negative consequences of behaving aggressively."[79] Imaging emotions is difficult enough when trying to comprehend the role of affect in healthy or normal populations, but the problem becomes even more complicated when assessing the relationships between potentially risky moods or feelings and psychopathology, as in the premise of the neuroscience of violence. Moreover, this example also speaks to the way expectations of the study groups inform neurobiological knowledges of violence.

Each clinical classification is thought to correspond to a unique brain response to these emotions. Thus, individuals characterized as psychopaths are supposed to express distinctive neural signatures compared to individuals who are diagnosed with a different personality disorder or condition. In the case of the neuroscience of violence, sometimes it appears that neuroscientists are suggesting a specific neural activation for violence, in which the "neural space" becomes a more distinct referent or unique signature of pathology. To illustrate, take the findings of one study on emotional processing in children with conduct disorder (CD). The neuroscientists conducting this inquiry found that *reduced* left amygdala activation in children with CD, compared to the study's normal population, diminishes the ability to recognize emotional stimuli that regulate, in cognitive terms, violence. That said, other neuroimaging studies have reported that *increased* amygdala activity for youth with

CD is what impacts emotional processing.[80] This implies that two different neural signatures—over- *and* under-active amygdala function—have been attributed to the same population.

Neuroscientists, to their credit, have indicated the need to better understand the delicate neurobiological differences that exist among behavioral traits for antisociality, such as aggression, callousness, and impulsivity[81]— although this has meant greater efforts to identify, or localize, specific functions of the brain into even smaller units of analysis. Such a move, however, may not solve this problem. Triangulating findings with animal studies or behavior studies, as mentioned by Dr. Smith, is another way to help neuroscientists be assured that their findings are valid. However, triangulation can "co-produce epistemological and ontological un/certainties, without wholly resolving philosophical and methodological questions regarding what mental disorders are, and how they can be recognized."[82] Thus, though it may be possible to observe and statistically link neurobiological correlates to a mental state, extrapolating the meanings of the brain's activity and mapping these findings upon traits for violence seem to require a set of assumptions or expectations that elude the technological capabilities of neuroimaging.

This critique is not specific to this one study or to the neuroscience of violence, but applies to social neuroscience research in general. As sociologist Gabriel Abend asks, "What are neural correlates neural correlates of?"[83] Abend pushes neuroscience to better attend to sociological and anthropological understandings to conceptualize phenomena of study. In the case of violence, however, the incorporation of sociological theory may present even more challenges given the primacy of macro- and meso-level social factors, conditions, and discourses that are central to sociological understandings of violence. It is more likely that the variable nature of violence, which is highlighted in social science conceptualizations of such behaviors, when filtered through the fitting process, will result in similar temporarily stabilized understandings, as seen with clinical definitions of antisocial behavior.[84] That is, truly attending to Abend's point involves going beyond the incorporation of social science literature, and opening up how connections among sociality and biology are meticulously erased, replaced, and reconfigured through the violent brain model; a construct that helps to transform any definition of violence into an already useful, and empirically truthful, set of neurobiological knowledges. Moreover, the aim to better outline neuro-correlates of cognitive or behavioral traits raises another interesting social fact, that in the process of creating data about study groups (i.e., participants thought to be at risk for violence), the violent brain model is also vigorously shaping neuroscientific perceptions of the normal.

THE NORMAL THROUGH THE VIOLENT BRAIN

Establishing normal populations for a study seems to be the other side of the fitting process. As demonstrated above, the violent brain model can help reassure classificatory boundaries separating antisocial, psychopathological, and other violent designations in research. However, examining violence through imaging also relies on a comparison group: a "control" population. Neuroscientists start their projects with the confidence that a *normal* or *healthy* brain is already a fact. That is, "the normal" seems to own an intrinsic value in neuroscientific projects on violence; the category's scope, meaning, and function are not discoverable, but already known before scientific or technological assistance. However, the making of the violent brain construct also assumes that there is a great deal of understanding of the "normal" brain in the first place, but this is not the case. During my interview with the neuroscientist Dr. Jones, I asked him to explain how the Jones Lab determines who should be in the control group for a study. He first responded that "establishing that someone is normal is usually easier than the converse."[85] However, as he went on, it became clear that the recruitment of a normal or control population is actually a much more complicated process:

> I just ask people to show up and then I see whether or not they have been violent or whether they have a psychiatric disorder. If they don't, they stay in the normal category, and that's all. We're taking all psychiatric disorders off the list. We're just taking normals, which means they have no Axis I, or in this case, also Axis II psychiatric disorders. It's actually very easy to recruit this group.[86]

First, these comments support an aspect that may be overlooked by those outside of the research: recruitment of healthy individuals is an essential task for the success of the experiment. As in study populations, there seem to be several tests or checks required of a "normal" individual before he or she is allowed to participate, the most important being that the individual does not have any preexisting psychological disorders or clear evidence of a history of violence. Moreover, Dr. Jones's statements demonstrate that this practice of imaging abnormal bodies simultaneously guides how "healthy" and "normal" populations should be made and realized. Thus, the normal brain and the pathologically antisocial brain are both "ideal types;" social constructs that are placed into relationship across this research, or more aptly, through an archetypal violent brain.

It is not really clear where or how neuroscientists draw the line between normal and pathologically violent. Beyond not having a psychiatric disorder, what does it really mean to have a normal brain, be a normal human being? That is, the normal or healthy brain seems to be just as elusive as the potentially violent one. In practice, a proper allocation of participants in the experiment implies that the study and control groups will be different enough that the data can be interpreted with certainty. Yet, this is not always the case, as one well-cited fMRI study on conduct disorder (CD) illustrates well.[87]

The authors of the study noted that the study observed between-group differences related to aggressive behavior in the ACC (anterior cingulate cortex) and the amygdala. While two groups in the study (one with conduct disorder and the other a control group) did show statistically significant within-group average difference in response rates for the experiment's task, there were also considerable overlaps in the results if we looked between groups.[88] Some individuals in the control group had identical, or similar, amygdala responses, neuro-signatures, as individuals in the patient group and vice versa.[89] The conclusions drawn here are not unlike those in other studies, where heterogeneity between the study's control group and target group cast some uncertainty.

Such struggles with navigating uncertainty may be less of a problem for experimental purposes, but when these scans (reflecting average differences between groups) are translated into other social worlds, like the legal system, they raise serious problems. One such problem, a heavily debated topic in the legal literature on expert testimony and neuroscience, is known as group-to-individual (G2i) interference.[90] G2i refers to the challenge of using scientific knowledge that has been derived from controlled studies as evidence in the courtroom.[91] It is unlikely that researchers can conclude conclusively that an individual on trial is antisocial or violent when comparing that individual's brain scan only to results from an existing study. The crux of this problem is that brain scans in published studies represent average group data, and therefore, are not a representation of individual brain function. Thus, the neurobiology of violent behavior is much more complex, and as mentioned throughout this chapter, experimental context and prior knowledge play a vital role in researchers' ability to properly interpret imaging data.

Psychiatrists have voiced similar concerns, noting that neuroscience research needs to pay greater attention to the way in which violence or aggression may be part of the "normal repertoire of human behavior" operationalized in their studies.[92] "The line between pathological and impulsive aggression and more normal forms of aggression is not hard and fast, and individuals with pathological aggression may experience or rationalize their violence or aggression as being within the boundaries of normal protective or defensive aggression."[93]

With each new advancement in the neuroimaging process, the focal point of the violent brain model shifts away from brains like that of the oft-cited Phineas Gage, and toward risky brains that more and more resemble what we think of as "normal" or "typical." Take, for example, a study that used a "mental imagery" task to help understanding of how the brain regulates aggression, and its relationship to impulsive tendencies.[94] Computer-assisted visual displays, strategy games, and creative storytelling have increased the potential of fMRI, and maybe the most interesting fact about these new tasks is that they often target *healthy* volunteers with no recorded history of antisocial behavior. In the study being discussed here, researchers first asked participants to picture themselves on an elevator with their mother and two unknown men. In the ensuing scenarios, the participants were asked to imagine one of three situations: (1) watch idly while the assailants attack their mother, (2) be physically restrained by one man, while the other attacks their mother, and (3) retaliate against the assailants, hitting them hard enough "to seriously injure or kill them."[95] The findings from the study noted that in imagined scenarios of an aggressive nature there was significant emotional reactivity and deactivation in cortical areas of the brain. The authors do note that their findings need to be replicated. However, my concern here is with the types of assumptions that are made about normal individuals or healthy volunteers, and the way the use of normal populations in studies of violence seems to also require the need for "docile bodies" during scanning.[96]

"Healthy" in this case was limited by one's imaginary abilities and compliance. The researchers said that participants all had "good or excellent visual imagery abilities and were trained in the experimental procedures to minimize anxiety or discomfort associated with scanning and thereby to enhance compliance during the study."[97] So not all "healthy" brains would have been suitable for scanning here. Additional exclusion criteria omitted volunteers if their parent(s) were deceased and also excluded those who had experienced any situation similar to the traumatic scenarios used in the experiments. The goal here seems to be to eliminate individuals who may have had social experiences or inabilities that might bias the results. Yet, the study seemed to overlook salient sociocultural factors that might have arisen during the research.

Specifically, these issues include how researchers were assured that aggression was the emotion that participants felt as a result of the scenarios, whether or not other brain areas could have been at play, if and how the magnitude of the emotion affected the participant's brain function; moreover, as the researchers themselves state, it would seem impossible to know for sure if the participants actually imagined one of the scenarios during scanning, and if so if they imagined the "right" scenario. Importantly, it is not clear what a "normal" response to "seeing" your mother attacked is supposed to look like. My point here is that the practical work of the violent brain model allows all of us to disregard or *forget* the social meanings and practices deeply embedded in the brightly colored, aesthetically pleasing images, and stabilize normative and authoritative assumptions about individual bodies and their (in)abilities to regulate their antisocial propensities. Lost, or normalized, within the making of violence into a neuroscientific question is the ability of biotechnologies to stabilize or reduce the sociocultural "noise" that is constitutively entangled in the making, expression, and management of these deviant behaviors in society. The colorful appearance of these representations for scientific and public consumption permits and perhaps sometimes implicitly encourages us to overlook the sociocultural meanings, negotiations, and omissions that go into the production of this work. That is, engagements with "pictures" of the brain sometimes inadvertently and sometimes by intention obscure uncertainties built into the neuroscience of violence.

Researchers may rationalize that such a study helps establish a baseline, a reference point for other studies to show that similar "normal" brain responses in, say, an antisocial group may reveal something about their aggressive nature. However, "it is not paradoxical to say that the abnormal, while logically second, is existentially first," as philosopher of science Georges

Canguilhem put it.[98] That is, we come to know what is "normal" or "healthy" through our engagements with, or socialized acceptance of, the abnormal. This point readily supports the chapter's larger argument that the violent brain is situated to produce and impel the neuroscientific interpretations that underlie these findings. Here, we find that the normal and its relation to the pathological are less a biological fact than indistinct notions whose value cannot be separated from their social purpose, which has important implications about the certitude afforded to neurobiological factors for violence.[99] Expanding to normal populations, then, has meant that the neuroscience of violence no longer needs to depend on pathological groups alone, which bestows a slightly different, but further empowering feature of the violent brain, to explicate the "at-risk" within any population. To be clear, I am not saying that the measurable distance between healthy and violent research subjects, which is so vital to the violent brain model, has shrunk. Instead, I am arguing that such an empirical space never truly existed. In producing a "picture" of the brain, or the violent brain, neuroscientists have also constructed a specific image of human beings, a potential *criminal* and seemingly simple and accurate representation of the *normal*. Furthermore, in Chapter 4, we will again see that neuroscientists try to address some of these concerns through the use of genetics, as a way to better type and apportion their "normal" populations and demonstrate the social nature of this brain-based understanding of violence.

PART II

THE UNMAKING OF THE VIOLENT BRAIN

4 | BEYOND DETERMINISM?

THE COMMON PERCEPTION of the biology of violence is that it produces biological deterministic claims about violent and criminal behaviors. For some time now, however, proponents of the research program have asserted that researchers never truly rejected social contributions as factors in violence (although it is evident that they have struggled to demonstrate this fact). Lombroso, for example, was said to hastily add other causal "social" factors to his larger theory of atavism when faced with criticism.[1] Race, gender, epilepsy, and even the weather (seriously, the idea that crime increases with the rise of temperature) were all additional causes that Lombroso made room for in his theory.[2] Frequently, the incorporation of these new factors weakened his position by illuminating the biases and inconsistencies in his theory. "The fact that Lombroso altered his original views to take account of social factors implies that the criticism that was leveled at him . . . may have led him to realize that his original theory was untenable," opined sociologists Alfred Lindesmith and Yale Levin in their 1937 article in the *American Journal of Sociology*.[3] They went on to describe Lombroso's explanation of social factors as "chaotic and confused."[4] Still, the flexibility demonstrated through Lombroso's *Criminal Man* theory is arguably one of his most lasting impacts on the program. It demonstrated the need for researchers to expand and rework their theories using the critiques leveled against the program. Moreover, there is also evidence that some, in seemingly antithetical disciplines, were persuaded by what we may call today a "biosocial" import of the program.

Just a year after Lindesmith and Levin's critique of Lombroso, sociologist Arthur Fink would conclude his review of the biological causes of crime in the nineteenth and early twentieth centuries, with the following: "We stand ready to conceive of the criminal as a biological product as well as a product of the environmental forces around him."[5] More than Lombroso's acknowledgment, Fink's review suggested that the program already regarded the underpinnings of violence as a product of the intertwined relationship between social factors and biological factors. He argued that the research program's "integrated personality" framework was the most optimal way to understand criminal behavior in society. This gesture to the biosocial echoes the sentiment of modern scientists and criminologists in the latter parts of the twentieth century.

Nearly two decades later, when Hans Eysenck provided his version of the biology of crime, he used the term "interactive" to describe the interplay between "inherited conditionability" (biological) and "lived environments" (social).[6] Around the same time, a similar view of violence was also being contemplated in the brain sciences. "No human behavior whatever, be it normal or abnormal, can be the consequence of the brain alone without the environment," stated neurosurgeon Vernon Mark in defense of psycho-surgery treatment for violent behavior.[7] In a similar fashion, contemporary neuroscientists who study violence contend that society's pursuit of an ef-fective answer to violence will fail unless the effort takes seriously the way neurobiological influences accrue meaning and significance through their interface with environmental factors. While this declaration hardly solves the elusive nature-versus-nurture conundrum that sits at the heart of the contentious debates about the biology of violence, it does provide a more robust platform for researchers to challenge their critics who are, in their view, hindering a *complete* understanding of violence in society. As discussed below, the idea of "completeness" involves an inherent belief in the ability of researchers to capture, calculate, and demonstrate the intersection between biological and environmental factors through neuroscientific *and* genetic understandings. Researchers believe that misunderstandings of biology, specifically genetics, among laypeople are behind the continued charge of biological determinism against the program.

Neuroscientists, like geneticists, uniformly reject the idea that the gene, or genetic contribution, is synonymous with a destiny of violence. Dr. Fitzpatrick expressed this position well during our conversation about the way neuroscientists respond to critiques of biological determinism:

> The main concern revolves around those knee-jerk reactions to the word "genetic." A common objection or misunderstanding is that people hear "genetic" and they infer that you're trying to have a deterministic account of individual violent acts, right? So, if it's a gene, then you can't do anything about it. You try and make people understand that this is not about predicting or explaining individual violent acts, which always arise from a very complex interplay of, you know, biological-biographical situations and factors, by clarifying a biological contribution, which in itself is also *quite minor.*[8]

Nevertheless, if neuroscientists do believe that the genetic contribution to violence is "quite minor," they have dedicated a substantial amount of effort to examining this lesser contributor to violence, particularly through investigations of gene-environment interactions. Here, the gene becomes another rubric to capture the way biology, through environmental influences, fosters *risk* for antisocial behaviors. Nevertheless, a (neuro)genetic-environment reading of violence has its own biopolitics, which have not necessarily been recognized or worked out, even as neuroscientists eagerly adopt and trust this epistemic in their daily research practices. As sociologist Thomas Lemke writes, "The thesis that biological factors play a role in the analysis of social and political behavior is not the problem; the question is, rather, how the interaction is understood—and in this respect the responses of biopoliticians are not at all convincing."[9]

GENETICS, VIOLENCE, AND THE MOLECULAR TURN

It was no accident that researchers studying violence at the end of the twentieth century turned to new genetic techniques. Earlier attempts to identify a genetic cause of violence had flopped, further fueling charges that the research program was at best "pseudoscientific." However, things began to change in the 1960s, when a team of geneticists reported a link between the chromosomal "abnormality" XYY and aggressive behavior.[10] For a brief period, the XYY research on crime was one of the most influential theories in the program. Although the original study focused on aggressive behavior, some proponents went further by suggesting that individuals with an extra Y chromosome—called "super-males"—had an inherent predisposition for criminality.[11] Furthermore, the "super-male" criminal narrative was reinforced through legal decisions, news reports, and popular media creations.

In 1968, Laurence Hannell was acquitted of murder by reason of insanity in Melbourne, Australia. The case drew worldwide attention after Hannell's lawyers argued that his compromised mental health was due, at least in part, to his XYY genotype.[12] Some scientists at the time questioned whether his genotype had any impact, however. For example, Allen Bartholomew, a forensic psychologist involved with the trial, along with geneticist Grant Sutherland, argued that Hannell's extra Y chromosome likely played *no* role in the jury's decision.[13] Later, however, Bartholomew seemed to support the idea that XYY genotypes are innately distinct, scientifically provable, criminal types. After the trial, he reportedly said, "Hannell has an extra Y chromosome additional to the normal male, which means that every cell in his body and the brain is abnormal."[14] Hannell's case was one of many XYY defenses during this time, prompting one *New York Times* reporter to write: "The evidence today may neither clinch the validity of the syndrome nor convict all the world's estimated five million XYY's of innate aggression or criminal tendencies. There does, however, seem good reason to keep an eye on it—and them."[15]

Shortly after, British author Kenneth Royce's 1970 novel *The XXY Man*, which went on to debut as a British television series of the same name in 1976, also helped to expand the reach of these narratives.[16] The fictional tale *The XXY Man* focused on an ex-felon who, despite his efforts, could not give up his antisocial tendencies, due to a predisposition for crime arising from his XYY genotype. Therefore, as in other courtroom accounts of biology and violence, the impact of XYY evidence functioned in a more discursive fashion in the larger public, seemingly confirming latent links between biology and violence as proven fact. The problem with both the legal and the popular translations of the XYY syndrome, however, was that the scientific research was much less conclusive.

Subsequent research efforts repeatedly failed to establish a definitive link between XYY and inherent criminality. There were mixed results suggesting that those with XYY genotypes may be more likely to display aggressive, and sometimes criminal, behavior, but these variances often disappeared once other (social) factors were controlled for.[17] At best, however, most studies could establish only that those with the XYY genotype were taller on average and possibly exhibited compromised intellectual abilities.[18] XYY defenses in courts also collapsed under scrutiny. In *People v. Tanner*, for example, California's appellate court upheld a prior decision to preclude XYY testimony in the criminal court. The court argued that XYY research was not precise enough to be used as evidence. While the research suggested a link to aggressive behavior, the court rightly noted that not all individuals with the genotype exhibit aggressive traits. Justices also questioned how scientists could truly prove that an individual's "chromosomal imbalance" was the cause of that person's aggressive behavior or, more fundamentally, whether the chromosomal condition satisfied the court's own definition of legal insanity.[19]

Few scientists today would regard the XYY argument as holding any sway.[20] However, historian of science Sara Richardson states that, "While the association between Y and aggression had taken a hit with the declines of the XYY hypothesis, the concept of the Y as the biological kernel of maleness survived."[21] The focus on the sex chromosome Y is guided in part by another seemingly natural fact about gender: having a Y chromosome is itself a (proxy) genetic predisposition to violent behavior. "We have probably already found the genotype that, in a statistical sense, predicts violent crime better than any gene to be discovered in the future. This is simply an XY genotype," opined psychologist Gregory Carey and behavioral geneticist Irving Gottesman in an article warning against the influence of "reflexive, knee-jerked medicalization of behavioral genetics" on public policy.[22] Carey and Gottesman's position carries an uncritical assumption about gender and behavior that needs to be examined.

Researchers in both the social sciences and the biological sciences agree that there is a "highly gendered ratio" in terms of crime and violence.[23] Yet Carney and Gottesman's use of the term "predicts" must be understood in a larger sociological sense, not as individual acts of violence. Gender differences in crime and violence are a product of larger social, not biological, facts and artifacts regarding the performance and utility of violence in society. More than a characteristic of identity, masculinity is better understood as a relationally conditioned and practiced response to specific social dynamics, and/or a privileged and productive extension of existing social hierarchies.[24] As criminologist James Messerschmidt puts it, "Crime [and violence] by men is not simply an extension of the 'male sex role.' Rather crime [and violence] by men is a form of social practice invoked as a resource, when other resources are unavailable, for accomplishing masculinity."[25] The usefulness of gender as a predictor of violence, then, rests on a recognition of the way such behaviors function in society as an effective, and often pervasive, practice of social power and control, and not simply a naturally induced inclination for brute force.[26]

Gender also becomes important for our understanding of biology and violence because of the presumed link between violence and the sex hormone testosterone. Research on testosterone levels has been presented, often dubiously, as an unquestionable source of higher levels of aggression, and therefore a key predictor for higher prevalence for violent or criminal acts.[27] Moreover, such logic does not always need to be explicitly stated. Illustrations of this "zombie fact" can operate in a seemingly benign fashion, as sociomedical scientist Rebecca Jordan-Young and cultural anthropologist Katrina Karkazis argue.[28] Jordan-Young and Karkazis persuasively illustrate that much of the scientific research on testosterone fails to question the cultural authority of "T," and how both scientific and social conceptions axiomatically equate the hormone to maleness.[29]

VIOLENCE AS A HERITABLE TRAIT

Around the same time that XYY research was facing intense scrutiny, the growth and sophistication of heritable studies of violence provided a more promising attempt to understand genetic contributions to violent behavior. The promise of twin, adoption, and family studies rested on the ability to illuminate and estimate a genetic contribution of violence *and* effectively tease out its influence from environmental factors. Twin studies of criminality compare the behavior between identical twins (monozygotic, MZ) and fraternal twins (dizygotic, DZ) reared in similar environments with the idea that any observed differences between the sets of twins indicate a unique genetic contribution—meaning that if MZ twins demonstrate a greater likelihood for criminal behavior than DZ twins, the variance is assumed to be purely genetic in nature. Moreover, this was exactly what researchers claimed. Twin studies reported that MZ twins have a higher concordance rate to crime than

DZ twins, meaning that MZ pairs exhibited criminal tendencies at a higher percentage.[30] However, as geneticists themselves point out, methodological and theoretical problems also frustrate the biological meanings revealed in twin study results. Thus, these findings are not straightforward.

Critics point out that MZ twins, due to their identical appearance, may actually have a more similar environmental experience than DZ twins, and that any observed concordance to criminal activity for MZ twins could just as likely have an environmental basis. Psychologists Sarnoff Mednick and Jan Volavka note that twin studies of violence may overestimate concordance percentages of MZ twins.[31] Instead of dismissing heredity studies, however, Mednick and Volavka claim that adoption and family studies are more informative methodologies, as they are thought to capture a cleaner separation of environmental and biological factors of violence. Adoption studies focus on children born to "criminal" parents who are reared in an adoptive "non-criminal" family. If the child develops criminal tendencies, particular at a higher degree than their foster siblings, then it is assumed that the variance is due to the child's biological predisposition to antisocial traits.[32] However, the way researchers define and distinguish "criminal" from "non-criminal" parents will affect the way the research findings are interpreted.

In the Mednick lab's Danish adoption study (one of the most famous such studies), convictions from official police reports were used as a sign of criminality. While conviction records may allow for a systemic allocation of study cohorts—children of "convicted" and "non-convicted" parents—official records cannot account for individuals who participate in criminal activity but avoid capture or prosecution. Adoption studies face a problem similar to that of twin studies concerning the assumption about equal environments; adopted children may experience different, and potentially unequal, social influences than their foster siblings do. Even Mednick and colleagues admit that "the relation between biological parent and adoptee criminal convictions exists at each level of adoptive parent SES" (socioeconomic status). SES does not fully capture the dynamic properties of "environment" that can also affect criminal convictions.[33] However, perhaps the most salient hurdle for researchers is the fact that heritability studies are, at best, proxy measures for genetic influence. It is impossible to prove that the observed biological finding is indeed genetic, nor can heritability methods alone demonstrate how or why genetics play a role in violence.

THE "WARRIOR" GENE

The promise to overcome this limitation came with the move to molecular genetics, an attractive option for behavioral geneticists who continued to struggle to legitimate their work on violent behavior as scientific.[34] Though the 1990s were identified as the Decade of the Brain, arguably the decade's most famous scientific venture was the ambitious Human Genome Project (HGP). Similar to technological developments now commonly tied to the rise of the modern brain and mind sciences, the focus on genes encapsulated larger technological advancements and an epistemological shift to molecular-level understandings of the biological world.[35] The HGP's goal to sequence the entire human genome, demonstrating the exact location of DNA sequences, sought to elucidate the molecular structure and function of genes, with the promise that such insights would help fully grasp and resolve a litany of diseases. However, the HGP and the Decade of the Brain were more complementary than antagonistic, as the focus on curing mental illness via the brain helped to carve out an avenue, scientifically and financially speaking, for geneticists to show how DNA could also help elucidate the foundations of psychiatric disorders and illnesses.[36]

Instead of merely providing estimates of trait expression of familial lineages, molecular techniques would allow researchers to identify the specific genes, and their properties, associated with violence and delineate how they work, i.e., demonstrate the mechanistic pathway from genes to violence. If violence is an inheritable mental trait, researchers argued, then its basis and function are coded in the structure of DNA. The first of such studies was published in the prestigious journal *Science* in 1993 by a team of geneticists in the Netherlands. "Evidence Found for a Possible 'Aggression Gene'" read the title of the journal's preview article for the upcoming paper.[37] However, the actual findings that Han Brunner's team published four months later did not quite live up to the announcement's latent hint of a direct genetic link to violence.

The group reported that impulsive aggression was correlated with a mutation on the monoamine oxidase A (MAOA) gene, an enzyme known to help break down neurotransmitters—chemical substrates that can inhibit or initiate neuron cell activity—such as serotonin. Similar to the heredity practices outlined above, Brunner's team traced the gene over four generations of men in one Dutch family; all the men in the family with the MAOA gene seemed to have some form of intellectual disability and a propensity for aggressive behavior—specifically, verbal threats and, in a few, physical aggression.[38] Combining these methods with advancements in genetics, the researchers found that all of the males in this particular family had reduced MAOA activity, an indication that their brains may not have been metabolizing serotonin properly, which possibly affected their ability to control their behavior.[39] However, as Brunner himself argues, the team's conclusions were not proof that MAOA caused these men to be violent or aggressive, or that MAOA was, in fact, a gene for violence. Brunner cautioned:

> The possible association of the MAOA deficiency state with abnormal behavior may contribute to our understanding of the pathogenesis of these behaviors. It does not, however, provide an easy explanation for them, and any causal link between the genetic defect and the behavior will involve several other factors, including some that are entirely environmental.[40]

Although Bruner continued to push back against crude interpretations of his lab's research, the paper set off a wave of new projects looking to further elucidate the genetic properties and connections between MAOA and violent traits in both human and animal populations.

More definitive proof of the intergenerational transmission of this causal link between MAOA activity and aggression was said to be confirmed in mice by researchers who used a genetic knockout technique later that decade.[41] In humans, stronger correlations were found when scientists focused on specific allelic variations of MAOA. Upon examination of differences in the expressions and enzymic activity between higher expression (MAOA-H) and lower expression (MAOA-L), researchers found that males with the MAOA-L variant were more likely to act aggressively and violently.[42] The focus on specific variants also led to a more serious attempt to take up Brunner's call to think more closely about the relationship between MAOA and environmental variation.

The first, and most well known, of these studies was completed by Avshalom Caspi and colleagues, who uncovered a gene-environment link between MAOA and childhood maltreatment. They reported that maltreated males with the MAOA-L variant had a higher likelihood of antisocial behavior and violent crimes.[43] Importantly, the Caspi et al. study also reported that maltreated children with a high variant of MAOA (MAOA-H) did not have elevated risk scores for antisocial behavior. Thus, the paper was also one of the earliest gene x environment (GxE) studies to imply that genes may act as a vulnerability for some and in turn perform a "protective role" for others—seemingly blunting the impacts of unfavorable environmental influences. Findings from follow-up studies have been mixed,[44] but the Caspi et al. study is still one of the examples most frequently cited to confirm the link between genetics and violence. This, however, has not been the case for many of the other projects that have looked at the role of MAOA-L, a result clearly demonstrating that controversy remains surrounding MAOA, specifically with regard to biological determinism and scientific racism.

Not too long after the publication of the team's paper, the MAOA gene received a new name, the "warrior gene."[45] This distasteful moniker emerged after the publication of a 2004 review article in *Science* reported findings from a team of geneticists that traced the evolutionary history of MAOA to a "monkey ancestor" millions of years ago.[46] The article, "Tracking the Evolutionary History of a 'Warrior' Gene," marked the first time the term "warrior gene" was used to refer to MAOA.[47] The name persisted, appearing often in popular magazines and newspapers, as well as in academic articles. Just a few years later, however, the "warrior gene" would be mired in a new controversy at the complex intersection of science, culture, and race/ethnicity.

The controversy erupted in 2006 after a group of geneticists presented findings that were said to demonstrate a higher incidence of the low variant of MAOA in the Māori population of New Zealand.[48] More specifically, the group found that the MAOA-30bp-rpt, an MAOA-L variant, was present in 56 percent of their Māori study population. While the work of authors Rod Lea and Geoffrey Chambers confirmed previous findings from MAOA-L research, they found themselves in the midst of a backlash after the New Zealand media ran a story highlighting their findings that the "warrior gene" was associated with aggressive tendencies in Māori populations. After the controversy that developed with regard to the study, Lea and Chambers caution against reading too much into the findings of their paper:

> [W]e reason that the MAOA gene may have conferred some selective advantage during the canoe voyages and inter-tribal wars that occurred

during the Polynesian migrations and may have influenced the development of a substantial and sophisticated culture in Aotearoa (New Zealand). It is important that the incidental formation of this "warrior gene hypothesis" is interpreted for what it is—*a retrospective, yet scientifically plausible explanation* of the evolutionary forces that have shaped the unique MAOA gene patterns that our empirical data are indicating for the Māori population . . . *negative twisting* of this notion by journalists or politicians to try and explain non-medical antisocial issues like criminality need to be recognized as having *no scientific support* whatsoever and should be ignored.[49]

While it is true that some journalistic reports of scientific research mischaracterized results, there seemed to be no need for "negative twisting," given the authors' own words. Thus, the cultural damage to the Māori population was already done. Lea and Chambers's caution concerning the misuse of their work does not sufficiently capture the more subtle and systematic ways in which the relationships between racialization and violence are often reconstituted and intensified through biological research. This defense, and the continued use of the "warrior gene" label, "reflects scientific and political convenience" that is misleading in both the bioscientific sense and the social scientific sense.[50] Moreover, such an interpretation leaves little room to explore, or explain, just how MAOA expression shaped, or was shaped by, environmental factors, seeming to suggest, even without genetic interpretation, an apparently natural evolutionary affinity for "warrior-like tendencies and characteristics" in this population.

"[I]f it turns out that low MAOA enzyme activity puts an individual at risk for a variety of mental illness[es] (and socially inappropriate behaviors) that are not necessarily related to violence, this interpretation may be inappropriate."[51] And this is exactly what neuroscientists have argued—that the prospect of using MAOA as a predictor of crime is limited because the effect size for the gene is low, and it seems to be involved in several different psychological disorders. As neuropsychologist Joshua Buckholtz and neuropsychiatrist Andreas Meyer-Lindenberg candidly point out:

> The current portion of MAOA suggest[s] that what it predisposed is not a specific behavior (violence) or set of behaviors (antisocial behavior), but rather a broader pattern of emotional dysregulation that can, but does

not necessarily overlap with these. . . . The fact would seem to seriously complicate genetic prediction of antisocial behavior and violence, as no individual maker would ever come close to the phenotypic selectivity that would be desired of a biomarker.[52]

Buckholtz and Meyers-Lindenberg state very plainly that due to these limitations and the fact that the gene has been implicated in multiple neuropsychological disorders, MAOA should not be used as a biomarker for violence. A recent meta-analysis published in the prominent journal *Molecular Psychiatry* agrees, noting that it is unlikely that this gene can be used as a biomarker for violence. In fact, the study found that the association between aggressive or violent behaviors and any of the twelve candidate genes in the study, including several polymorphisms of MAOA, was weak at best. This result led the authors to conclude that "aggression and violence exist on a continuum that makes it more likely that they are determined by many genes of moderate or small effect."[53]

Genes, then, are less certain in this new configuration of violence, and that undistinctive characteristic essentially undermines the current value of molecular genetic studies of violence, especially the hope that such research will yield a distinctive biomarker for violence.[54] However, uncertainty also serves an ethical purpose, as it helps demonstrate that the future of the gene goes beyond the pitfalls of biological determinism. This point was made clear in my conversation with neuropsychiatrist Dr. Jones:

> I don't see egregious things being done around me in terms of this research. You know, like people making claims based [solely] on genes. I don't see much of it. But [some scientists] did participate in a [PBS] *Nova* episode, "*Can Science Stop Crime*"? Which is a stupid question to begin with, right? But even there, one of the scientists talked about the "warrior gene," which was a bit too—I'm usually more careful when I interview with the media.

Dr. Jones went on to argue that the most realistic goal for the science was to demonstrate the complexity in various manifestations of violence.

> [That scientist] was looking at his own brain scan and saying that he has the warrior gene, but he is not aggressive so . . . [However,] it was good

because he shows that it's not enough to just have that gene. I mean, forty percent of men in the United States have the warrior gene. It doesn't mean that they're aggressive. Not at all, actually. And then you have people who are very aggressive who don't have that gene. So, the picture is a complex one, and I think that's the message that most scientists convey.

Using the MAOA gene alone as a marker for violence can lead to an overestimation of violent individuals, a false-positive. Genes, then, become one of the first links in the attempt to outline the potential that an individual is at risk for a personality disorder, which would then place that person at greater risk to engage in violent behavior—ostensibly a risk for riskiness. However, other factors must also be taken into account, and even then, researchers will still have a difficult time assessing which individuals in the estimated 40 percent of the population who have the gene will be violent. Aware of these limitations of genes, neuroscientists turn back to the brain to better assess risk.

BIOSOCIAL DESIGN

In his 1977 presidential address, American Society of Criminology president C. Ray Jeffery urged fellow criminologists to adopt a new biosocial direction in criminology: "Sociologists deal with age, sex, ethnic background, and urban areas as major correlates of crime rates. These are viewed as social variables, whereas a little reflection will reveal that they are biological and social variables. There is no such thing as a social variable; there are only *biosocial* variables."[55] In essence, Jeffery's comments should also mean that there is no such thing as a biological variable of crime, either, and the absence of this comment, and ostensibly the unique privilege afforded to the biological here, demonstrates the unsettled contentions that undergird, and at times undermine, the push to replace sociological criminological perspectives with biosocial ones.[56] Similar to Jeffery's remarks, the biosocial emphasis in the program today has tried, although at times haphazardly, to push back against determinism by recognizing and incorporating social/environmental factors into the research on biology and violence. As one interviewee noted:

People are paying a lot more attention to biological-environmental factors in psychiatric conditions. And I think there's very few psychiatrists you can talk to who would say, "Oh, it's just men, or it's only the genes."

> Anybody that's read the literature in the last few years—anytime in the
> last ten years—knows that it's not just the genes. It's not just the environ-
> ment. *It's both.*[57]

It is pretty much an axiom that neuropsychiatrists no longer say "it's only the
genes," as today's researchers reframe their work in terms of gene x environment (GxE) interactions, in which the interplay between *both* biological and
environmental factors is used to help make sense of a studied phenotype.
However, what's not always clear is what these two sets of factors mean. In an
attempt to provide conceptual clarification, one group of researchers detailed
the logic they use to define social and biological variables. They defined "a
variable as 'biological' when it reflects a biological measure of a biological
construct. . . . Similarly, [they] define[d] a variable as 'social' when it reflects
a social measure of a social construct."[58] If this seems overly simplistic, that's
because it really is. Social/environmental factors seem to imply anything
that is not a biological measure—standard demographics, environmental
stressors, diagnostic variables, or even psychological or cognitive features.
Moreover, the idea that these *two* forces, broadly biological and social, are
intersecting can also be limiting in practice.

Technological advancement was supposed to replace an "additive" biosocial approach—biology in addition to a social variable explains violence. This
view was indicative of biosocial attempts in the past, which were biosocial
in name, but most of the scientific focus and even sociocultural significance
rested on a very static and authoritative role of the biological variant.[59] In
its place, the molecular revolution was supposed to provide a more comprehensive, technologically driven take on the way these two seemingly
disparate factions affect each other. This was the significance of the Caspi
et al. MAOA article. Neither the MAOA variant nor child maltreatment
alone could produce the outcome that was observed when the group thought
about the way the interaction between two variables influences the risk for
antisocial behavior. However, even the interaction here was not that the biology and environment worked upon *each other* (a fuller way to capture
possible *interactions*) but that the MAOA modulated how and when child
maltreatment mattered for the phenotype. And, as mentioned, replications
of the study findings were not always consistent, a potential result of the
variability in definitions of social notions like "child maltreatment," but also

an indication of the difficulties with recognizing and elucidating a truly *integrated* influence, which would seem to suggest a bi- or multi-directional impact. Thus, it still is not clear that these models are actually able to achieve such interactional complexity.[60] Dr. Hollowell noted in our interview that at best, this is still a work in progress:

> We are really taking a more comprehensive look at biology by looking at multiple things at the same time as well as looking at what we used to think of as just environmental variables, trying to put everything together. That's been happening more and more. It's still hard to put things together, completely, but we're definitely moving more and more down that road.[61]

This biosocial logic derives from an examination of two distinct variables for violence, albeit intersecting in one fashion; the emphasis above on "It's both," meaning genes *and* environments (not genes and biosocial variables) makes this clear.

Despite Jeffery's claim, then, that social variables are really misinterpreted biosocial variables, neuroscientists are still needing to identify and define each social variable separately, and then tease out how it may act on the biological variable. "The first thing you want to do is see if any of these factors bear any relation to your main measure. So, if it's aggression or some biological measure, you want to make sure that a [social variable] does not influence the data," Dr. Hollowell explained during our conversation.[62] Thus, a "biosocial" variable for violence does not naturally exist. Instead, "biosocial" is a product of research design.

The meeting of genetics and neuroscience makes clear that the two contemporary biological approaches to violence are not necessarily distinct disciplinary fields. Researchers rely on their recognition of, and access to, the interplay between genes and brains to authorize their calculations of risk for violent or antisocial behavior.[63] Neuroscience and genetics practices are "*thought-styles,*" joined through a shared technoscientific specificity to produce a seemingly less rigid, more useful vision of violence. Turning to the brain has, at least in theory, helped smooth out some of the limitations of GxE interactions.

The brain, or brain functioning, is thought to best capture the molecular-level effects of GxE interactions. To be sure, this move is not a simple substitution of gene facts for brain facts. Instead, neuroscientists and geneticists view it as a logical experimental direction, a combining of insights from molecular genetics with the violent brain model. As Buckholtz and Meyer-Lindenberg put it, "MAOA biases brain development toward alterations in function and structure that are associated with individual differences in personality that may predispose, in combining with other factors, the development of antisocial behavior."[64] In terms of the neuroscience of violence, this picks up where Caspi's group left off, re-situating MAOA through its role on the brain. Thus, the true scientific import for the genetic variants is best realized through its complex expression on the violent brain model.

In a related manner, neurobiological substrates operate as a third factor in the etiology of violent behavior, reflecting an acknowledgment by neuroscientists that they "sort of have to study a social context"[65] to dispel the deterministic moniker, and make an explicit nod to the violent brain model, especially its bestowed authoritative power to help overcome complexity. Essentially, a crucial value of this construct is its presumed amalgamating function that unites the operation of the gene and experiences of social environment within the brain. The social context is conquered by the brain or, put differently, the nature-nurture divide is now "bridge[d] by the brain," according to neuroscientists.[66] The program's contemporary biosocial vision of violence, then, is inextricably linked to the function of the brain.

Neuroscientists, therefore, must design their methods and questions to be meticulous enough to pick up the trace of these "interactional" properties. Practices related to actualizing the violent brain influence researchers' ability to interpret how and where to see and engage with the social, i.e., where biosocial-ness is at work. This is often as much about the social insights that were gained through the fitting process, such as choices made for types of social/environmental factors that will be measured and how, or the expected ways these variables are thought to matter for the brain. As a result of this move, the program is better situated to outline the biosocial importance of the knowledges produced through neurobiological models, and to defend its position concerning the discourse of completeness, that brain understandings fill the gaps in knowledge left by social scientific, humanistic, or legal understandings alone. Neurobiological understandings of biosociality, then, are not necessarily intended to supplant current (meaning sociological or legal) understandings of violence, but instead are privileged as a missing data key needed to *complete* the view of violence. The completed view of violence is interpreted through the notion of risk, and especially *vulnerabilities*.

DISCURSIVE VULNERABILITY

In this biosocial view of violence, the violent brain model is the tool that helps neuroscientists pick up and interpret when and how biomarkers for violence are activated, or exploited, by social causes. Vulnerability immediately directs attention to risk, thus reminding critics that such language should not be mistaken as an endorsement of biological determinism. As Dr. Jones said, "Just because you have a vulnerability to something doesn't mean you're going to get it without, you know, the *right* environment problems."[67] This reference to the "right environmental problems" indicates the discursive quality of vulnerability that is at play when neuroscientists are assessing the value of environmental forces acting on the gene. In this sense, the knowledges yielded here can reflect multiple and flexible conceptions of vulnerability, all fitting into a seemingly shared value spectrum in the field: favorable, right, and positive on one end, and harmful, adverse, and negative on the other.

For example, some interpretations attempt to follow vulnerability as it travels from the gene to the brain, a process thought to grasp the way certain environmental influences on the gene exposes brain function and structure to risk:

> Genes code for proteins that influence characteristics such as neurocognitive vulnerabilities that may in turn increase risk for antisocial behavior. Thus, although genetic risk alone may be of little consequence of behavior in favorable conditions, the genetic vulnerability may still manifest at the level of brain/cognition.[68]

The idea that neuroscientists believe that biological vulnerability may present in multiple ways on the brain, should not be surprising. Biological vulnerability is similar to the arguments in Chapter 3 that the presence of certain biomarkers may appear differently during imaging, and thus require some form of intuitive reasoning (i.e., the value of functional differences in an at-risk individual may work differently than the detection of imperceptible structural differences). Thus, there is a need to extract value, the right kind of value, of environment to help decipher when vulnerability matters for violent behavior.

Exploring genomic approaches to autism, and especially the "molecularization of environment," sociologist Martine Lappé shows how the maternal body is transformed into a genetically valuable variable through flexible conceptualizations of environment. Through the "molecularization of environment" here, the transformation of the environment happens at a more discursive level. Certain types of exposures become more vital to the biology of violence, but just as important, so do certain kinds of populations. Therefore, the molecularzation of environment obscures "political and economic conditions that structure the unequal distribution of exposures."[69] A similar process can be observed as neuroscientists try to make sense of the value and role of environment through the violent brain. As these narratives of environment, and their relationship to individuals, are sifted through the violent brain, understandings of social environments are conflated with static readings of personal experiences, thus obscuring the more dynamic and unequal structures that help make and manage such social contexts.

Take, for example, what is sometimes called the "social-push hypothesis" for antisocial behavior.[70] In this hypothesis, the moving from "genes to brain to antisocial behavior"[71] suggests that biological markers may explain less of the variance for violence for individuals who come from social environments that "push" them toward risky or violent behaviors. In other words, if an individual from a more "negative" environment engages in violence, the cause may be due more to social environment than to genetics.

The social-push theory acknowledges the various and complex ways in which social factors can influence violence, yet this understanding also seems to dictate how the researchers should value the social environment. A specific sociocultural value is attached to vulnerability here, in the sense that environmental risk is equated to "negative" environments. My point is not to dispute that unfavorable life chances can be correlated with violence: there's little debate that "maltreatment" can influence a child's likelihood to engage in antisocial behavior. And, in essence, neuroscientists are acknowledging that social factors may be more important explanations of violence for certain individuals.[72] However, there's a noteworthy normative presumption here, which suggests that the behavior of someone from a more "positive" environment is *less* significantly affected ("pushed") by their social circumstances. That is, if someone from a more-privileged background commits an act of violence, then the cause that is more easily understood, or at least empirically proven, is inherent neurobiological dysfunction. Social environment, here, becomes entangled with, and seemingly substituted for, a more comprehensive understanding of social experience.

Not all neuroscientists refer to this hypothesis as "social-push," but there is evidence of a similar logic. As one neuroscientist stated to me:

> It's a yin versus yang kind of thing. The stronger the biology is, the less environmental stuff you need and vice versa. It's very much kind of a balancing act between biology and environment. Basically, if you're really healthy, it's going to take an awful lot to get you sick. If you're not as healthy, it's not going to take very much to get you sick.[73]

One consequence of using clinical terms to illustrate environmental differences is that health is correlated not only with a positive environment, but also with a normal one. Thus, the normative position here establishes a link between normal environments and anticipated normal experiences. Individuals matching these criteria have a particular usefulness for neurobiological experiments, as their social and environmental factors allow researchers to deem them normal, or more-normal, individuals. This reasoning builds upon the discussion about the importance of normal populations beyond the control group. In neurogenetics, a person designated as normal—that is, lacking a known psychiatric diagnosis—becomes an ideal candidate to illustrate the unique influence of biological factors on violence.

> One way to try to start and disentangle those various contributions to violent behavior is to look at one of them in isolation. And so, that's what imaging genetics are doing, looking at people who are completely *normal*; in particular, they're not violent in any sense or fashion. They are different in either having or not having a genetic variant that has been associated with a disposition towards violent behavior. What you're doing in these studies is that you take a bunch of "normals" who are otherwise fine, so they don't take medication and have not been incarcerated. They don't differ in their socioeconomic status and so on. And then what you're doing is looking at their brain structure and functioning using your imaging. Then you stratify people by genotype and whether or not they have this variant that's been associated with violent behavior and see

if you see any difference. If you do, given that you're controlling for most of the other confounding factors, you're beginning to make a case that that system is what is active in the brain *to the presence or absence of that genetic variant.*[74]

Vulnerability, or the lack of it, opens up an avenue to better isolate biological factors. The importance here is not just that environmental experiences act differently upon genetics, but that they are manifested differently at the brain level. If more challenging environmental measures, like low SES or maltreatment, mask the effects of biomarkers, researchers' ability to disentangle the biological contribution from the social cause of violent behavior becomes more difficult.

Demonstrating the underpinnings, and therefore the potential, for violence in a normal population goes a long way toward expanding and explicating a more comprehensive theory of risk. However, social experiences cannot be neatly equated with social environment, nor do social advantages and social privileges (i.e., social experience) invalidate the social as an explanation for antisocial behavior. Measures for environmental influence represent only one way, or at best a few ways, to think about the relationship between the body and the social world. However, there are multiple interactions, memberships, and meanings that continually work upon and through our bodies that help make social action.[75] Thus the operationalization of the vulnerability process also seems to reinforce very specific configurations and values of the gene-environment relationship that engender, or at least preserve, specific biopolitical and social assumptions as well. The point is not to undermine the attention to the social in today's neuroscience; rather, it is to question just what the social is and how it matters, beyond "a reflection [of] a social measure of a social construct"[76] whose significance is realized through very specific techniques for reading the brain. Moreover, the concern here is not just what counts as "favorable" or "unfavorable," but how neuroscientists link these inferences into a tenable empirical vision of violence.

BIOSOCIAL COMPLETENESS

While society has spent the majority of its resources thinking about sociocultural influences, proponents of the biology of violence suggest that the model will never be complete as long as biological factors are neglected.

When considered in conjunction with the notion of biosocial, the discourse of completeness is rendered necessary, yet flexible, logic to understand all the factors involved or for treatment purposes. For example, genetic evidence is seen as "necessary for a more *complete* understanding of the transmission of violence from one generation to another."[77] Although having a parent or sibling who is violent does not guarantee a future of violence, "completeness" here infers that genetics provides the missing data needed to solve the hereditary puzzle of violence. Similarly, others have drawn upon this discourse of completeness in clinical settings. A 2012 *British Medical Journal* article by a group of physicians urges fellow physicians to take advantage of their unique opportunity to diagnose the symptoms of clinical violence.[78] In their words:

> When manifested as domestic abuse, road rage or workplace violence, [violent] behavior is commonly attributed to cultural factors, social stress, economic deprivation, or substance abuse. Much more needs to be known about these behaviors; however, recent advances in neuroscience allow for a more *complete* understanding, which accounts for biological factors amenable to medical treatment.[79]

In this medicalized view, "completeness" refers to the discovery of biological points of intervention, genetic pathways that can be targeted to improve the efficacy of treatment for violence. To understand how the discourse of completeness operates on and through the violent brain model, we need to take a slightly broader view.

The crux of the completeness discourse for the violent brain rests on the logic of multicausality. First, there is a presumption here between causality and certainty, in the sense that fulfilling this causal chain of "genes to brains to antisocial" in an experiment will yield the right answers for violence. Meaning that the idea of "incompleteness" already has a schematic ordering (its "biosocial design") that neuroscientists seek to follow. By knowing that genes will inform *how* the social will matter, and *what* social will matter, and by filtering through the violent brain, neuroscientists are convinced that they have captured how these "integrated" forces affect risk.

Similarly, neuroscientists have prevailing assumptions about what is "missing" and why it's important. As a result, biological components are privileged as necessary, but unaccounted for, factors in these models. Yet, just as there are multiple biological factors and systems that can be examined, there are just as many social influences and mechanisms that affect violence. For social scientists, a multicausal picture of violence may contain only factors that can be described as social or cultural in nature, yet this description may nevertheless be deemed *complete* in that specific field. Thus, it is not that completeness is an objective, or agreed-upon, course of action, but it is a course of action that is thoroughly embedded within the imaginary of a particular research program or discipline. In this case, completeness reflects the ideal set in motion by the violent brain construct.

The meaning or look of completeness in practice, then, is hard to pin down. While strategically employed as a critique of non-biological or non-biosocial meanings of violence, its own significance in neurobiological models of violence is just as elusive. In fact, technoscientific improvements have not necessarily provided greater understandings of complex disorders, and it is not really clear if or when neuroscientists have reached a *complete* understanding; these models are always in the making, always in process, more so than they are conclusive. Sociologist Stefan Timmermans makes a similar point in his ethnography of genetic labs: "Geneticists face the paradoxical situation that even though they have access to information about more genes than ever before, it becomes also more difficult to establish causality due to uncertain, unknown, or anomalous findings."[80] Timmermans finds that these scientists have, interestingly, abandoned complexity for more simplified explanations, yielding a "narrow causal narrative where one gene corresponds to one or more traits."[81] Part of this slippage back to the older conceptualizations of genetics has to do with the disappointments with molecular genetics. While molecular genetics was supposed to save behavioral genetics, Aaron Panofsky writes, "molecularization failed to quell the field's epistemic problems or quiet its controversies."[82] This "failure" of molecular genetics led many geneticists to return to the older claims from behavioral genetics, which "become a relative oasis of certainty and consensus as molecular genetics produced ambiguous results."[83]

Uncertainty and complexity seem to prevent complete biological models. This is supposed to be the work of the violent brain, to iron out these complexities and to sanitize these models to rid them of uncertainty. However, very similar to the genetic models (which are folded into a neurobiological understanding of violence), the violent brain model has not been able to fully remove these obstacles. Its true function, then, is to provide more of a way to instill the conviction that these models are *more* complete than others. The multiplicity of factors analyzed through practices of the violent brain—including the continually shifting fitting process, helps to reassure neuroscientists that their conceptualization of violence is not only correct, but *more* correct than models that do not include neurobiological influences. However, the idea that multicausality yields a complete model of violence is much more of an ideal than a reality.

Neurobiological models have limits on what can be included. There will always be decisions made about what is measured—and, importantly, how it is measured (fitting) and made meaningful throughout the process of the violent brain. Rarely have the questions, findings, or recommendations from the biology of violence reflected the richness and candor evidenced through its researchers' appeals for biosocial appreciation. The research program's historical silence toward, and at times vigorous encouragement of, policies that promoted questionable medical treatments, scientific racism, and eugenics laws speak well to this point. Today's researchers of biology and violence acknowledge this past, yet quickly reject the idea that either their science or they themselves would support such horrific outcomes, given the current use of more-superior technological practices and a firmer adherence to a biosocial framing. However, even as today's researchers continue to call for a biosocially complete understanding of violence, the insistence among advocates that social factors do matter is often undermined by the continued need to explain, rationalize, and justify the program's ability to truly deal with sociological experiences.

Social/environmental measures that are used in these models of violence are often limited to very specific, quantifiable, and seemingly non-partial factors. Problematics of violence, like race, gender, and social power—which often serve as exemplars by critics of the program's insensitivity toward sociality—present too much complexity for these biological models of behavior, and therefore are avoided altogether. To be clear, I am not saying that the biosocial framework employed here is insincere. I believe scientists when they say that social variables have to be taken into account to appreciate the etiology of violence. However, when critics of the research program talk about violence as a social construct, they are not simply speaking to singular social factors that relate to violence. They are drawing attention to the powerful dynamics informing how society reacts (rationally or not) to individuals labeled violent, and they are pushing back against the idea that the "violent" and the "non-violent" are clearly distinguished social identities or easily demarcated social experiences. These continual warnings against the misuses or abuses of biopolitical regimes challenge the need for translation of social traits into calculable biological differences that readily utilize, if not reauthorize, existing modes of social power and inequality.

5 | THE TABOO OF RACE

IT IS IMPOSSIBLE TO TALK about the social consequences of the violent brain model without examining the program's turbulent history with race—specifically, its function as a "racial project" throughout much of the twentieth century.[1] Lombroso's initial conception of the "born criminal" was made through an image of race, as he asserted in the final chapter of *Criminal Man*, "Those who have read this far should now be persuaded that criminals resemble savages and the colored races."[2] Such racist propaganda made his work particularly attractive for policy-makers in places like the United States, who were eager to embrace a "scientific" vision of crime that aligned with existing racial politics prevalent throughout the U.S. South *and* North.[3] In a similar fashion, elements of the research program can also be found in Nazi practices during the 1940s. Although the biology of violence did not directly produce such policies, its underlying contentions that crime is the result of inferior genes and that "medical" solutions to crime exist did influence the Nazi regime's eugenic practices of sterilization and extermination.[4] Following World War II, however, there was a shift in the conversations about race and biology, spearheaded by the famous UNESCO statements on race in the 1960s, which extended to the biology of violence, shaping how its psychological rebirth would address the question of race.[5]

During this period, the program's fixation on race was substituted for supposed racialized traits of violence like mental ability, emotions, and intelligence. Such proxy variables do similar racial work. Instead of tying race directly to innate criminal propensity, the measure of such traits acts as a mediator between race and crime. For example, a lower IQ score was emphasized as a key reason for increased rates of criminal behavior, and unsurprisingly, low IQ was said to be an innate characteristic of some racial groups, like African Americans.[6] In this sense, racist tenets of the program remained after its midcentury return. However, there were greater, or at least more noticeable, consequences for scientists who produced this bias research.

Hans Eysenck, who help initiated the return of the program after World War II, tarnished his prestigious career after coming to the defense of his former postdoctoral researcher Arthur Jensen's controversial research on race and intelligence. Eysenck largely repeated Jensen's flawed claims, arguing that heritable genetic factors best explained the gap in IQ scores between whites and blacks.[7] In defense of his apology for scientific racism, he wrote: "I am not a racist for believing it possible that negroes may have special innate gifts for certain athletic events, such as sprints, or for certain musical forms of expression. . . . Nor am I a racist for seriously considering the possibility that the demonstrated inferiority of American negroes on tests of intelligence may, in part, be due to genetic causes."[8] This defense is directly tied to a common trope of racial science: the assumed "right" for the public to know the true facts about a given phenomenon, even if the results are unpleasant. Around the same time, however, a separate group of neurologists proposed a much different biomedical approach to violence, which initiated its own unique racial controversy.

The group claimed that violence was the result of a neuropsychological illness that could be cured through a surgical procedure called *psychosurgery*, essentially a lobotomy.[9] The procedure promised to identify defective brain areas thought to cause the illness, and through the proficient removal or destruction of such lesions, alleviate unhealthy behaviors or emotions associated with the illness.[10] However, three years before the publication of their book *Violence and the Brain*, Vernon Mark and Frank Ervin, joined by their colleague William Sweet, set off a public controversy with an article they published in the prestigious *Journal of the American Medical Association* (*JAMA*). The trio's editorial brief argued that "urban riots" may be caused by a brain illness or, as they wrote:

That poverty, unemployment, slum housing and inadequate education underlie the nation's urban riots is well known, but the obviousness of these causes may have blinded us to the more subtle role of other possible factors, including brain dysfunction. . . . The real lesson of the urban rioting is that, besides the need to study the social fabric that creates the riot atmosphere, we need intensive research and clinical studies of the *individuals* committing the violence . . . to pinpoint, diagnose and treat those people with low violence thresholds before they contribute to further tragedies.[11]

The authors faced heavy criticism from colleagues and other academic professionals, and the Letters to the Journal section of *JAMA* became one arena where this debate played out.

Citing his own clinical experience, forensic psychiatrist and former president of the American Academy of Psychiatry and Law Seymour Pollack replied, saying that violent rioting could not be explained as a brain disorder.[12] A year later, Mark and his colleagues responded to Pollack's comment, insisting that their original article was meant only to be "an appeal to suspend judgment [of the cause of urban rioting] until enough facts could be collected by intensive research and clinical studies of the individuals committing the violence to warrant an answer."[13] However, this reply failed to address Pollack's larger point. He described personal observations with patients who had very similar brain lesions but did not express violent behavior; thus the presence of lesions alone was insufficient to explain the cause of violent behavior. Pollack cautioned that a narrow focus on brain abnormalities encourages a misdiagnosis of normal behaviors as violent behaviors, which was even more dangerous given the fact that psychosurgery is irreversible.[14] Intriguingly, critiques of the racial undertones embedded in the claims about psychosurgery played out in a separate journalistic arena.

The popular African American magazine *Ebony* became an alternative forum for professionals and the public to voice their concerns and, in a sense, speak more directly to the African American community. In the February 1973 edition of the magazine, Harvard psychiatrist Alvin Poussaint is quoted as bluntly stating:

[Mark and colleagues'] study is racist, it assumes that black people are genetically damaged—that they're so animal and so savage that whites have to carve on their brains to make them into human beings. The whole concept is vicious. When all these institutions around the country decide to study violence, who do they go look at? The *black* man. But who's committing all the violence? The *white* man, white society, white policeman [*sic*]. They don't consider that something's wrong with *their* brains. . . . [This research] is a spin-off from the old genetic theory, which held that blacks commit crime because of inferior intelligence.[15]

Poussaint was right. He stressed that there were no clear medical or scientific guidelines in place that could distinguish with certainty violent behaviors from normal behaviors. More importantly, he made clear that the argument put forth by Mark and his colleagues lacked a convincing neurobiological warrant for the study of black "rioters." They failed to justify why an organic brain disease explanation was deemed suitable for describing the cause of rioting in the midst of the social turmoil of the 1960s, but *not* the extreme violent behaviors of law enforcement or political officials against marginalized groups during this era.

Moreover, Poussaint felt that this "treatment" for violence would actually further empower racist state-level policies and practices that would further engender and reinforce social control. As acclaimed poet and activist James Baldwin poignantly noted in response to a question about the pervasiveness of violence in the United States toward African Americans during the 1960s, "The [U.S.] is only concerned about non-violence if it seems that I'm going to get violent. It's not worried about non-violence if it's some Alabama sheriff."[16] *Ebony's* subscribers shared Baldwin's position. As one replied, "These doctors are, as is clear from the article, primarily concerned with individuals 'involved in any uprising such as Watts or Detroit,' and that means any black person who is not prepared to sit back and meekly accept the grudging hand-outs from the white man, and who has no other recourse but to fight for justice and his [*sic*] self-respect."[17] Such worries about the strategic and racialized use of this brain model of violence against African Americans who were publicly protesting for civil rights were certainly plausible, given the way that psychiatric professionals had misused their authority to target and diagnose protest behavior as a mental illness during this period.[18] Thus the warnings to African Americans were clear: this line of research would only bring greater surveillance, criminalization, and oppression to their community.

MAKING A "COLOR-BLIND" DEFENSE

The debate in *Ebony* was so influential that Bertram Brown, then director of the National Institute of Mental Health (NIMH), penned his own reply in the magazine's November 1973 issue. Brown tried to assure the public that he, and therefore NIMH, shared many of their worries. He stated that NIMH would initiate its own ethical review of psychosurgery to help assuage African Americans' concerns about the procedure.[19] Around the same time, both Mark and Ervin wrote new commentaries in *JAMA* to again explain the rationale of the 1967 article. Mark responded that while there are political implications of the theory, such implications do not suggest that brain-based violence is an inherent characteristic of African Americans like Eysenck's IQ theory of crime.[20] Writing later that year, Ervin conceded that police officers did in fact cause many of the violent deaths during the 1960s riots and that the majority of victims were African Americans. Ervin's larger point, however, was to argue that critiques of psychosurgery were misunderstanding the dynamic nature of violence. He contended, instead, that the groups' true aim was to spotlight a rare subpopulation of individuals who exhibited "episodic dyscontrol," a symptom of a mental disorder characterized by the absence of impulse control, which is still recognized today as "intermitted explosive disorder."[21] Apparently, the focus on "urban riots" was just a way to bring attention to the disorder. Ervin declared that the 1967 article poorly explicated the researchers' true intentions, but also wondered why anyone would believe that their article proposed that *"riots* were a product of brain disease or that *rioters* were to be accounted for by the presence of medical abnormality."[22] Contrary to his shock and disbelief, however, the article did suggest that rioting by African American protesters was a symptom of an underlying mental illness, and therefore it was more than fair to question its racial overtones.

By the late 1970s, scientific and popular debates just about ended the chances that psychosurgery would be accepted as a legitimate remedy for violence. Fears of scientific racism was not the only reason for its fall, but it was certainly a key factor. For example, activism and legal action from social justice groups, like the Black Panther Party, helped stop the development of a national center on "violence and the brain" at UCLA that would have been headed by Frank Ervin.[23] Significant to our discussion about the violent brain, Mark's and Ervin's rebuttal arguments vis-à-vis race foreshadowed an emerging strategy toward the delicate topic over the next decades.

In making the claim that their research was not intended to target a specific racial group, the neurosurgeons argued that their work was inherently *color-blind*. As Mark opined in his 1973 piece on the social and ethical issues of psychosurgery:

> In my experience, there is not a special correlation of violence with race. . . . It may be very well that violence in ghettos more often gets reported in police records and other data available to the sociologists. But the perspective of the physician is the emergency room and clinic where the products of violence are immediate. *From this perspective, claret is the predominant color, not black or white.*[24]

First take note of how this comment suggests that "the physician" has some unstated advantage in understanding the causes of violence. The hospital or clinic, apparently, represents a space in which the troublesome social milieu can be suspended, allowing physicians to understand the "immediate" causes of violence. Color-blind biomedical approaches, like this one, may seem impartial, but they threaten to silence the historical and contemporary racial effects engendered through biological logics of difference.[25] These approaches insist that the best way to deal with racism is by disregarding race altogether, meaning they deny the continued effects of race in society.[26] This view restricts racism to very explicit individualized forms of prejudice, or renders racial dynamics an offshoot of more-significant social forces such as social class, culture, or ideology.[27] The new form of racism that emerged in the latter decades of the twentieth century would be accented by the preservation of "racism without racists."[28]

Assessing the "success" of Mark and his colleagues' color-blind approach during the 1960s is difficult. They clearly failed to convince the public that their original claim about rioters lacked any racial undertones. Yet the import of this rhetorical move can be understood by examining how today's neuroscientists wrestle with the historical trappings and lingering residue of race when trying to construct their image of the violent brain. In its contemporary form, this color-blind tactic operates as a strategy that I call the *taboo of race*.

THE TABOO OF RACE

In its most straightforward interpretation, the taboo of race represents an inherent sociopolitical response to the research program's historical legacies with regard to race. As an infrastructural component of this science, the taboo of race is an informal, yet normalizing, reconfiguration of the policies and practices that help order and produce contemporary paradigms of the violent brain. This strategy is evidenced in several ways: an absence of the topic in research publications, trepidation when working with race in lab practice, and fear of discussing race within public *and* professional spaces. Therefore, as a sociological analytic, the taboo of race helps to illuminate how the program's historical struggles with race are embedded within and realized through the making of the violent brain construct.

The haunting past of race in biological research on violence acts as a constant reminder to the public and neuroscientists alike of the racist and deterministic origins of the biology of violence. There are, however, some who disagree. Behavioral neuroscientist Diana Fishbein, for example, warned that being captive to the program's past will inhibit the promise of neurobiological research on violence. In Fishbein's words, "Critics argue vehemently that biological research must be seen in the context of our racial history or racial attitudes. . . . Defenders of the research, however, deny that it must be captive to our racial history, and argue that it will ultimately do far more to *alleviate* than exacerbate racial tensions."[29] It seems that for Fishbein the best way to move past the program's history of scientific racism is to leave it in the past. However, acknowledging an awareness of the turbulent racist, and sexist, history of biological research was commonplace for the neuroscientists I interviewed.

Among those who agreed to participate in the project, many felt more comfortable steering questions about race toward a historical context. "I am aware of past problems. . . . I think all young scientists are aware of the history of aggression research," one neuroscientist told me when I asked for descriptions of the potential impacts of race on the research. However, the troubled history often served as the starting point and the stopping point of this discussion. It took more work for them to open up about complexities of race in their own projects. And when they did talk about race, they seemed to configure the violent brain as a "race-natural" project. A close inspection of the standards and best practices of this science demonstrates how racial meaning can readily be inserted into discussions of the making of the violent brain. Thus, contemporary attempts at erasure have led only to an "absent presence" of race.[30]

"Absent presence" has a normative and methodological function, "oscillating between reality and nonreality, which appears on the surface and then hides underground," according to social scientists Amade M'charek, Katharina Schramm, and David Skinner.[31] The *effects of race*, then, are woven into both the production and the potentialities of certain scientific knowledges. Attending to the function of the *taboo of race* reveals the strategic points of absence making, as it helps in interrogating the actual work, standards, and articulations of researchers' attempts to "deracialize" contemporary paradigms of the violent brain.

To be clear, the neuroscientists that I spoke with had no desire to construct a white, black, Latinx, or any other racialized (or ethno-racialized) reading of the violent brain. Yet they seemed unable to address the way racial meanings are implicitly built in and concealed through the making of the violent brain via formal and informal policies and research protocols. Moreover, the taboo of race is explicitly practiced during conference proceedings, training, and classroom lessons, as well as engagements with the public. As Dr. Moore described it during our conversation, "The (neuro)scientific community tries to be scientific without, you know, looking too much into race."[32] The consequence is that "not looking too much into race" most often materializes in studies of the violent brain as ignoring the impacts of race altogether, a *race-neutral* logic.

THE "UNSAID" AS RACE-NEUTRALITY

Combing through nearly thirty years of published peer-reviewed journal articles on neuroimaging and violence reveals a conspicuous absence of the term "race." In his ethnography of PET imaging labs, Joseph Dumit observes a similar treatment of race in published PET neuroimaging research, noting that measures for race are employed inconsistently or eliminated altogether from the analysis in order to minimize confounding effects.[33] At first, this obvious omission of race appears to substantiate the idea that today's research program is more progressive than the racialized depiction of the "diseased" protester's brain from Mark and his colleagues. However, the absence of race actually tells a different story. Published research on the brain and violence is not as much totally devoid of race as it is sanitized of meaningful discussions about the impacts of race.

Over the same thirty-year period, medical and public health experts have pushed to reform the way biomedical research deals with social difference. No longer should the 35-year-old white male be the only standard of research. Instead, major state-sponsored agencies in the United States, like the National Institutes of Health (NIH), abandoned the "one size fits all" research and initiated concerted policies that help recognize and include an adequate representation of social groups.[34] As mentioned in Chapter 2, a good number of neuroscientific studies on violence are financed through national, government-funded agencies like NIH, or their equivalents in other countries. NIH requires statements about the collection of racial and ethnic categories, and justification if a project is not using an inclusive sample. Nevertheless, when race (or ethnicity) is mentioned in neurobiological studies of violence, it is often limited to demographic charts.

Here it seems that the main function of collecting data on the race/ethnicity of populations is to produce racially/ethnically congruent research groups. Racial congruency here refers to the methodological practices that try to mirror the racial/ethnic identities of study and control groups. Racially congruent research samples can help minimize the chances that unexpected (or unmeasured) social factors will bias the study's outcomes and control for racial-based differences in findings. Controlling for race in this way is not necessarily a deliberate attempt to sidestep the issue of race in biomedical research; social scientists also employ the method to make sense of race in statistical models. Sociologist Tukufu Zuberi, however, illustrates plainly that these accepted methodological practices do not do enough to capture the dynamic significance and power of race within our society, or its impacts on the practices and production of scientific knowledge.[35] Thus, reducing the effects of race to a variable that merely outlines groupings and/or mediates differences in research outcomes misses the way that racial interactions and experiences influence the makeup, occurrence, and evaluation of violent behavior. Dorothy Roberts refers to a similar process in genomic science as the "statistical erasure of racism," which prevents researchers from engaging with the dynamic sociopolitical salience of race.[36] In the case of neuroscience research on violence, investigations that limit race to a demographic descriptor, while scientifically sound, can obscure the mundane and inherent impacts from complex sociocultural racial biases and anxieties and the way such social forces can influence their own scientific decisions and outcomes.

Controlling for race also illuminates more than methodological tactics. As Dr. Smith noted,

> Now we certainly would never speculate about the role of race in any of our findings. We just kind of leave it unsaid. Now, I suppose it's possible that people reading the research assume that if we're studying kids with behavior problems, that these kids in our studies are black. But, I don't know. Does that mean I should state strongly that the variables that we're looking at are race-neutral, which they are as far as we can tell, I don't know. It's tricky.[37]

Dr. Smith's comments illuminate the other concern: leaving race "unsaid." Not clarifying the racial, or potentially racializing, impacts of the variables used in this research opens the door for others to read race into the violent brain model and raises important questions: What actually counts as a race-neutral variable? How can others know that the measures identified in this research are race-neutral? The fact is, most researchers sidestep these questions, as if neutrality has no politic. Adherence to neutrality misses the way color-blind understandings operate through practices of rationalization, and therefore absence gets equated with the progressive ethic of the program.[38]

The function of race-neutrality, then, is driven as much by the goal to provide a more socially productive science as by an insecurity with race and, more than often, an anxiety to resist the label "racist scientist." This is a vivid example of the way color-blind logics of the social world are intimately entwined and reconstituted through the making and rationalization of neuroscientific knowledges of violence. What this means is that scientific dealings with race are not unique, but rather a reflection of society's own dealings, and misdealings, with the "weight of race."[39] The taboo of race, in this instance, elucidates the methodological difficulties and potential repercussions from race-knowing or -thinking within biological models of violence. And, in doing so, it shows the (in)abilities of neuroscientists to articulate the powerful ways in which race produces and affects conceptions and actual manifestations of violence within their research.

WHERE (HOW) TO TALK RACE?

Race-neutrality is supposed to reduce the chance that neuroscientists produce biased or misguided understandings about violence. In addition to race-neutrality, the neuroscientists who participated in this study would interpret my inquiries about the impacts of race as questions about *racial differences* in research outcomes. Dr. Hollowell, for example, talked about the sense of discomfort about whether the lab's findings might indicate racial differences in aggressive behavior. To the question "How do you think your research is perceived in relation to race?" he replied:

> You know, I don't know how my work is perceived around the issue of race, because I haven't reported any race issues. It's not like I've written any papers saying, "aggression is more likely in blacks because of serotonin levels that are more abnormal in blacks than whites." I don't have those kinds of findings, so hopefully people will not think of my work in those terms.

Dr. Hollowell works with adult populations diagnosed with personality disorders associated with aggression. The combination of the lab's study location and its advertisement strategies has enabled the research group to recruit racially diverse populations, according to Dr. Hollowell. So the reply that "hopefully people will not think of my work in those terms" speaks to a specific fear, that the lab will have to report or explain differences found between the groups.

> DR. HOLLOWELL: We don't think there's any race thing going on here. We do think, however, it is probably some socioeconomic factors, and certainly educational factors [influencing the susceptibility to the disorder]. And certainly, younger people tend to be more susceptible than older people, but that's kind of expected. . . . And let me tell you something. I'm glad I don't have those findings.
>
> ROLLINS: What type of findings do you mean?
>
> DR. HOLLOWELL: I'm glad we don't have any findings that show [racial differences].

To be clear, I too am glad that Dr. Hollowell's lab does not have "those findings." Dr. Hollowell is probably right that differences will be filtered through existing racial ideologies, which will likely reinforce negative stereotypes about the group. However, differences, in this sense, do not speak to why and how racial groups may have diverse findings. Moreover, the dread of racial differences seems to arise from the need to protect the researchers, labs, and discipline from unfavorable political or public backlash. Thus, the taboo of race seems to help erect invisible boundaries that structure how the violent brain is made and designed to be used.

Academic classrooms, for example, are a space that permits discussions about race, racism, and differences. However, many such discussions are limited to understandings about the history of race and biocriminology. In Dr. Smith's words:

> I feel like the questions that you are asking about race are really interesting, but a lot of researchers will be *extremely* reluctant to address them at all. For me, I think of the really racist historical events that have happened as not too distant history, and I actually teach about them in my classes. I teach a class on the social impacts of research on aggressive behavior, and I certainly teach undergrads about how important it is to not fall prey to older assumptions [about race and aggression]. I talk about the history of believing that there are racial differences in aggression, you know?

Discussions of race in the classroom—a seemingly less political, if not productive, environment—give the perception that race may be less of a problem for today's researchers. This may not be an accidental change. Debates or questions about the contemporary impacts of race are scarcer in other social spaces related to the program. Dr. Smith also made this point:

> So, I talk about race quite a bit with students, but I don't bring it up as often in professional talks, mainly because it's such a loaded topic, you know? Again, a lot of people are just afraid of addressing questions about [race].[40]

It is telling that the more *public* conversations about contemporary impacts of race—such as those that take place at professional talks—have remained taboo. Professional talks could be a space in which neuroscientists try to address racial anxieties, yet here again we see the absent presence of race. While I am sympathetic to Dr. Smith's efforts, the problem is that limiting conversations about race to classroom history lessons for students does not do enough to address adequately the contemporary social and ethical implications of race on today's research. The difficulties of having such conversations about race with colleagues cannot be solved by avoiding the uneasiness or awkwardness of the continued significance of race in our thinking about violence. In fact, not discussing issues or questions about race probably does more to extend color-blind forms of racism than it does to purge the program of its problems with race. Neither the neuroscience of violence nor the violent brain construct is race-neutral; thus not talking about race only sidesteps the actual and potential issues of racial bias, discrimination, or inequality.

Rather unexpectedly, another neuroscientist I spoke with revealed that such boundaries have also created a space in which curiosity about racial differences is more or less tolerated. Dr. McKinney suggested that the journal peer-review process can serve as a protected arena for neuroscientists to query racial differences in brain functioning. As he put it:

> No evidence that currently exists shows any major differences based on race, or even culture or gender, that we can pick up with fMRI. [And] if we do see any differences it is probably just *noise*.[41]

"Noise" refers to residual or unexplained variation that exists after running a statistical analysis. This is one of the justifications for controlling for race, or any other variable: to provide more-definitive results. Yet, as Dr. McKinney continued to talk, it became clear that the appearance of "noise" also signaled a curiosity about racial differences.

> The fact is, journal reviewers get very excited about [noise] and want us to tell them more about such differences, which we'll do, but we never find any [significant] racial differences.

Anonymity is the key here, as it seems to indicate a presentation of neutrality. Although such a request from peer reviewers may be common, it neverthe-less provides an alternative (and protected) channel to discuss race, which is noteworthy for a discipline that strives to present itself as detached from racial politics. Such discussions are, for the most part, protected under the banner of anonymity, well outside of the public's purview, and it may be that anonymous reviewers, who may or may not research violence, feel more com-fortable requesting information about race from anonymous authors.[42] A few other neuroscientists also noted that they had been asked to re-run analyses to further inspect potential racial differences, although it is not clear whether this also extended to other demographic lines, such as age, socioeconomic status, or sex. Nevertheless, Dr. McKinney's comments imply that the taboo of race ensnares the entire program, well beyond the lab work. In this way, race may be erased from methodological consideration, but it is certainty possible to capture its trace during the publication and presentation of the science.

ANYTHING BUT RACE

Another unintended consequence of the taboo of race is that researchers often reduce race to socioeconomic and/or cultural factors to arrive at better explanations of racial differences. Here, the role of the taboo of race logic is trickier, as such arguments rest on a valid assumption that race, as an individual attribute, has nothing to do with the "phenotype" of violence. Dr. Jones explained this position in our interview:

> You see, [neuropsychiatrists] have fidelity to the phenotype, and then all the rest we don't care. It's not that we don't care, but we sort of blindly look for the things that predict the phenotype of aggressive behavior. And, *the phenotype has nothing to do with race or even education or things like that*. [Instead], it has to do with very specific questions and very specific psychiatric interviewing, which does not ask about demographics or anything like that. So, I don't feel like [race] is an issue too much.[43]

Dr. Jones's comments return to, and substantiate, the role of fitting in the making of the violent brain model. Race is not a biological product representing an innate shared quality or character that can delineate clear and specific groupings or be mapped upon specific behavioral phenotypes, but sociologists have been clear that it a *social fact*.[44] Race is best captured as a fluid yet embodied social process, constructed through difference/power and realized, made meaningful, and reconstituted through social practices, institutions, and relationships.[45] Still, this does not dismiss the fact that phenotypes remain a powerful lens through which we engage with, come to know, and value race. Therefore, if we think about race as a social process, and not a variable, we also have to acknowledge that the effects of this social practice will certainly affect how the neurobiological sciences understand racialized behaviors like violence.

The logic of "anything but race" has meant that some researchers have dropped race in favor of seemingly more salient variables of difference. As demonstrated in the exchange below, some neuroscientists resist the use of race because they see other social factors, like class, as better explanations for social difference in relation to violence.

> It doesn't matter where you're from, men are men and women are women. There is no culture in the world that doesn't have a concept of male and female. It's robust. But, if we can't [evaluate] gender differences, something so universal that it cuts across all cultural boundaries, [then] we can't pick up differences based on race. We are not there yet. It's not that I don't believe that racial differences exist. I think, however, that ultimately, though, we'll find that culture plays a dramatically larger role than the actual genetic variances that make people appear one race or the other.

That contemporary neurotechnologies are too crude to capture racial or gendered differences is an important point. We should appreciate the acknowledgment of the impacts of social forces, and not just biological units, on the actual expressions of and perceptions toward violence. Nevertheless, by limiting explanations of difference to culture, neuroscientists are also implicitly closing off any discussion about race.

My argument, however, is not that culture does not play a role in violence. Instead, I am suggesting that because race, or understandings of race, are so narrowly construed through the taboo of race, researchers are more likely to downplay or overlook the existing and future racialized impacts of the violent brain. Translating potential racial differences into an expression of cultural differences minimizes the distinctive operation of racism and racialization. There are certainly ways in which culture affects differences in the rates of violence, but race and culture are often used interchangeably in a problematic manner, and such a conflation cannot be substituted for an antiracist stance, nor will it quell concerns about the science reinforcing scientific racism.

As exemplified in the exchange below, we can also see how the *taboo of race* does not necessarily prevent more critical thinking about race, at least for "violence" in general compared to the biomedical rendering that is supposed to occur through the violent brain. Dr. Lewis commented:

> Well, certainly, I think it's important to understand culture, race, gender—all of those different types of variables that might lead to differences. With respect to personality disorders [related to violence], however, I think that there's lots of evidence that says that they do not

discriminate. They're equal opportunist. . . . I think that the reason why there's such inequality in violence is because of socioeconomic problems and socio-demographic kind[s] of problems.[46]

Dr. Lewis's point was that there is no evidence that personality disorders related to violent behavior affect one specific racial (cultural or gendered) group more than others. This explanation comes the closest to grasping the role that sociological dynamics play on the production of violence. And while I agree that age, education, social class, and overall cultural factors are important for understanding the manifestation of violence, it is still unclear what is meant by "culture" here. Culture certainly operates in a dynamic fashion, through language, customs, signs, kinship or beliefs, which are often inseparable from the way racial identities are expressed and made meaningful in society. Still, sociologists make clear that race, racism, and/or the processes of racialization are unique social properties in their own right.[47]

Sociologist Janet Shim describes this methodological move as the *cultural prism*. In health research, the cultural prism captures when researchers neglect how race organizes social relations of power, and instead read racial/ethnic health differentials as products of the group's cultural values.[48] "Such practices can replace structured understandings of race with individualized ones that ignore the ways in which relations of power are embedded within the reciprocating representations of race and the material consequences [that] such representations have on life chances."[49] It remains unclear how neuroscientists will ultimately deal with these "relations of power," race or other; however, it does seem clear that a type of cultural prism works through the taboo of race as well.

Another important aspect about the use or race versus ethnicity has to do with location. The term "race" is often used more in studies of U.S.-based research, or research on U.S. populations, whereas "ethnicity" is preferred for research conducted outside of the United States (although I found that a few articles used the terms interchangeably). Part of this variation can be explained by the lack of a clear definition of race. Like social scientists and health researchers, neuroscientists will often use self-identified race as a way to indicate race/ethnicity. However, the concern here is not only a question of the way researchers define their populations, but how they understand and consider the salience of race. According to Dr. Lewis, who worked in both the United States and the United Kingdom,

It's very interesting that [race] is not something that's touched on particularly well in logical work at this stage. But, it's just too sensitive. For example, there was very interesting work concerning immigration and the effects of ethnicity and the over-representation of black and minority ethnic groups in British psychiatric systems, which all came from British data. This research wasn't the sort of thing that was looked at by American epidemiologists. So, there can be cultural biases operating at that level, concerning what types of research can actually be done.

Cultural differences between the United States and the United Kingdom that are alluded to here are in part products of racial politics that originated through historical power relations, contemporary social arrangements, and scientific (academic) knowledges that helped shape each culture's protean taxonomies of identity and sense of social difference.[50] Race and ethnicity are related but different concepts; to deny this specificity is to "blur the particular history by which these identifications come to have the force they do."[51] Shedding the shroud of scientific racism, then, is more complicated than simply substituting ethnicity for race. However, I also want to stress a key point in Dr. Lewis's reply: how the *effects* of race/ethnicity affect scientific research practices.

The notion of violence alone provokes its own unique racial/ethnic narrative, which already links particular racial groups, and representations, to violence.[52] For example, historically, young black men are often implicitly linked to notions of dangerousness or criminality. Similarly, the image of a "terrorist" has also been racialized and limited in a unique fashion, to Arab- and Muslim-"looking" men, a more recent consequence of the racializing culture. The impact of cultural racism is even more pressing given that there have been recent attempts to explore the neurobiological underpinnings of "terrorism" and "violent extremism." Interestingly, the neuroscientists who undertook such investigations have focused on identifying the parts of the brain that are active during "sacred values"; thus they do not view terrorism as a mental illness.[53] They do, however, suggest that scanning the brains of potential terrorists can help prevent future attacks. Contextualizing the work through contemporary social events, cognitive neuroscientist Nafees Hamid proposes that such data may yield important clues about the mind of the "next white-nationalist" attack.[54] Yet, it is difficult to imagine that this work will not help reinforce cultural stereotypes about "radical Islamist[s]," since all the brain scans are from "Sunni Muslim Moroccan [young] men."[55]

Academic and lay audiences often use race and ethnicity as proxies for inherent violent or criminal tendencies Just think for a moment about the representations of violence in U.S. society. What comes to mind for Americans when considering who is, or will be, a "violent offender," "a criminal," "a rapist," or "a terrorist"? None of these social descriptors of violence is racially neutral. In her analysis of identity politics, national security, and the perception of threat in the United States after 9/11, communications professor Kumi Silva writes that a new perception of "Brown" emerged, which was "not separate from the historical somatically defined deployments of color but instead [was] harnessed and extended to any behaviors, places, spaces and performances that challenged the hegemonic Whiteness of U.S. neo-nationalism."[56] Silva goes on to connect the racialization of Arab- and Muslim Americans to larger ideologies of insecurity and threat: "Because these deviant outliers challenge the notion of a particular and recently repopularized version of American nationalism, it was seen—and continues to be seen—as necessary to rearticulate those deviants as *a threat*."[57] Silva's emphasis on the historical, cultural, and political function of "Brown threat" speaks directly to the timeless Du Boisan question raised in *Souls of Black Folk*, "how does it feel to be a problem?"[58]

Racial identity, more specifically racial worth, actualizes and warrants a seemingly constructive societal politic to suspect, target, and surveil people from specific racial or cultural groups more than others not only for national and domestic security needs, but also to preserve, if not enforce, a particular racial ordering of society.[59] These racial politics are embedded within and realized through the larger dialectical operation and maintenance of identity politics, on the one hand, and the continued struggles for civil rights in the United States, on the other. In particular, the politics of race capture how the everyday practices and experiences of racial identity interact with, are navigated by, and are experienced through the impacts of systemic racism. Reducing the management of race to affirmations about the program's racist past or strategically erasing the visibility of race in printed publications cannot fully eradicate the immense weight of this sociopolitical force. In this sense, the paucity of attention on the politics of race in the neuroscience of violence, can unintentionally rationalize, and reconstituted, the seemingly practical linkages between violent behavior (potential dangerousness) and specific racial groupings that are stubbornly refashioned and extended through the dialectic of national insecurity and protection (safety).

FAILURE TO "SEE" RACIAL LIVES

It is too crude, and impractical, to perceive the neuroscience of violence as a neo-eugenics endeavor engineered by racist scientists. Neuroscientists' perceptions of race are complex and varied, and better captured by the efforts to inoculate the research program from racism through the adoption of a race-neutral approach to difference. Simply thinking about violence in socioeconomic or cultural terms does not mean that the influences of race, racial discourses, or racisms are muted. That is, the violent brain model is not immune to the tenacity of race just because the term "race" does not appear in print. Ultimately this speaks to a larger challenge: to think more critically about the biosocial associations, and more specifically about the consequential effects of race, particularly *racial living*, more than just race as a research variable.

Dr. Smith all but acknowledged this during our interview, admitting that an assessment of racism is indeed necessary in order to understand the underpinnings of violence:

> Because I'm looking at such incredibly basic, low-level, simple variables, I really don't end up spending a lot of time thinking about racism and those levels of complexity. I mean, we're just not there yet in understanding anti-social behavior. I know that there are interesting questions to be asked, but I don't feel ready to add that layer of complexity in my work yet. And it's not that [racism] is not important. I see racism as a covariant that is important to keep in mind, but not one that I have any theories about right now.

The complexity that evades Dr. Smith results from the lack of a more dynamic operationalization of difference; a missed opportunity to articulate how racism is experienced in relation to understanding of the risk for violence. Attending to the *effects* of race means recognizing how racism, racialization, and powerful sociocultural practices and institutions undergird the ongoing confluence of the politics, ideologies, and logics of difference that help police how life is lived, whose life is valued, and whose life is devalued.

So, the larger question, then, is this: *can* the violent brain model process how racial inequality affects our understanding of these behaviors? At least one group of neuroscientists has tried to answer this question. What has been notable about the work of neuropsychologist Luke Hyde and his colleagues is that they have named structural effects, like racism, as a driving factor for differences in observed brain activity. Thus, Hyde's work is not simply controlling for race. Instead, it is acknowledging the need to consider "African Americans' disproportionate exposure to low-income, dangerous neighborhoods," which the neuroscientists note are already used as predictors of violence, yet not conceptualized in most neuroimaging studies.[60] In a 2020 study on the biosocial impacts of socioeconomic disadvantage, Hyde's lab found an association between neighborhood poverty and activity in the inferior frontal gyrus, a brain region said to be linked to inhibition. The group noted that "the poverty level of a family's neighbors, may affect the developing brain and subsequent performance on a critical indicator of self-control."[61] Hyde's approach is rare, and most studies lack this level of conceptualization and analysis of race, as suggested by Dr. Smith's comments. Their research also utilizes the growing neuroimaging research on racial bias to help explain how social experiences with race likely give rise to observed brain differences.[62] However, the incorporation of this research may prompt more questions than answers.

There is neuropsychological evidence that the brain plays a role in our implicit associations about race.[63] Some of these neuro-knowledges are familiar, particularly the inability to control emotions and the role of the prefrontal cortex as a governor of unwanted actions and thoughts. How would scientists properly assess amygdala activation? Does it "light up" because of impaired emotional traits that reflect a risk for psychopathy or antisocial behavior? Or does it signal fear or hostility toward another on the basis of racial identity? For that matter, how do neuroscientists studying race differentiate these signals as well? Is this just left up to neuroscientific "intuition," as we learned in Chapter 2? Moreover, it is unclear how the violent brain model would make sense of implicit racism/racial bias, given that it cannot deal with the explicit impacts of racism, and the fact that it reads brain inabilities as biomedical symptoms working on more of a linear than relational plane, and in a quantified more than qualitative fashion. Either reading of the brain (as implicitly biased or neurobiologically risky) can—without careful attention—draw our focus away from the normative ways in which police officers are trained to detect who is and who can be a criminal. Neighborhoods do not just happen to be dangerous or impoverished, and African Americans are not simply being profiled, arrested, or murdered because they lack inhibition. I do not doubt that Hyde's group of researchers studying racial bias would likely agree with much of this statement.

Yet they may miss the fact that their own goals to elucidate the effects of race may actually signal the need for a shift away from a dogged concentration on individualized risk for violence and toward a more nuanced analysis of the way structural social experiences are inextricably bound to the way violence is perceived, policed, and researched in society. In the words of criminologist Darnell Hawkins, "Social researchers must not replace the quest or a measure of *real* crime with a renewed search for the *real* criminal.[64]

The challenge for any assessment of difference is to locate and make sense of the impacts of such attributes within the societal spaces that make meaning and structure experiences. For example, Shim calls for greater attention to the social relations of power, and the specific mechanisms through which inequality or marginalization is produced—that is, the social spaces that work between, and conceptually bind, our practices of identity and our experiences of health (or behavior).[65] Thinking about identity as a key discursive practice, Stuart Hall describes it as the meeting point, or *suture*, between these spaces, joining the subject to the structures of meaning.[66] Taking Shim and Hall together, I argue that it is not simply a question of *adding a layer of complexity* to the violent brain. Without accounting for the suturing effects of identity, the intricate relationship between *race* and *racisms*, the violent brain is rendered woefully unable to grasp salient social qualities and experiences tied to violent behaviors.

Thus neuroscientists are left wrestling with what Duster calls the "unenviable task."[67] That is, researchers must figure out how to effectively consider racialized experiences without "endowing race with a false sense of biological determinism," or contributing to and/or buttressing an individualized and racist justification.[68] I submit that this task will be complex and/or impossible given current neuroscientific tools, or quite possibly inimical to a research program seemingly trying to rebrand itself as indifferent to race. This, though, is the point. Nothing about race is simple or straightforward, but there is no doubt that its pervasiveness and embeddedness in society have normalized our perceptions and practices of violence and criminality through a "peculiar" tint of difference. Race itself is a *technology* that constantly innovates new *natures*, which obfuscate historical realities, reanimate inequities, and police futures.[69] Thus, if neuroscientists are serious about developing biosocial understandings of violence, they must deal with the way race not only stands in for identification, but also the way in which the making and management of such classifications become normalized, expected, and naturalized technologies to "see" and evaluate the properties of violence. This too may be difficult, if not impossible, for the violent brain in its current configuration, but that is the point.

The taboo of race makes clear that the violent brain has inherent racial vulnerabilities. If neuroscientists are unable to capture the complexities of racism, why then should a group, like African Americans, for instance, trust that this science will indeed benefit and not further subjugate them given the inadequate function of and discriminatory outcomes from the current systems of law or health. Such groups have even less of a reason to place trust in a science that has historically relied on mischaracterizations of marginalized and stigmatized populations to validate its worth in society, if there is no effort to understand how the effects of race continue to punctuate their lives. If the taboo of race is not taken seriously, then race will continue to trouble neuroscientists who will have to deal with the disproportionate ways that criminalization and racialization intervene in and operate reciprocally in society. Moreover, this perpetual haunting of race may be the loudest signal that the violent brain may be "trans-scientific."[70] In this sense, race will likely continue to be a question asked of science but will remain fully incomprehensible through this "color-blind" technology.

6 | FIXING VIOLENT BRAINS

AT THIS POINT, we return to a question raised at the beginning of the book: What does the violent brain model suggest we do about that toddler in the prison-striped onesie. That is, what are the potential interventions, or fixes, for those who are neurobiologically at risk for violence? Scientists have been reluctant to advocate biomedical interventions for violence since the return of the research program during the mid-twentieth century. Advances in technology alone, at least ostensibly, have not been able to fully soothe the scars that remain etched in our collective consciousness regarding the horrors of eugenic experimentation during the Nazi-led racial hygiene movement. The exception, as we saw in Chapter 5, was psychosurgery, which was once publicized as an expansive solution for various forms of deviancy, from individual-level criminal acts to racially charged notions of "urban violence." Psychosurgery cures for violence were not eugenics, but critics assured the public that they nevertheless carried a more subtle threat to society: "seek[ing] not to discipline through punishment but to rehabilitate or remake through treatment."[1] Overall, the potential for a psychosurgery cure for violence quickly rose and then fell during this time.

Interestingly, however, the curiosity of the larger public about a biomedical cure for violence would remain, sustained in part through influential cultural resources, like science fiction. For example, one of the most popular science fiction depictions of brain science gone wrong is Philip K. Dick's 1956 short story "Minority Report"—and the 2002 blockbuster film of the same title that was based on the story. The plot centers on a futuristic governmental agency, the "precrime division," which was developed to identify and arrest would-be criminals before they engaged in criminal activity. The novelty of the precrime division rests in the abilities of "precogs"—a select group of individuals with extraordinary psychic powers, although otherwise described as incoherent "minds [that] are dull, confused, and lost in the shadows."[2] When precogs are hooked up to "analytic machines," law enforcement officials are able to capture and decipher their psychic visions through "computing mechanisms" that yield the names of those soon-to-be "criminals."

Neuroscientists are not secretly developing a "precog" system to arrest individuals before they commit a crime. Yet the dystopian future portrayed in "Minority Report" is relevant for this discussion because it helps contextualize the continued interest in a technological fix for violence. Today's scientists do hope to predict, but in contrast to the precogs' seemingly certain image of criminals, the violent brain model describes susceptible individuals who, under less predictable and unfavorable situations, might be unable to restrain their behavioral impulses and act out violently. Nevertheless, working in terms of brain risk instead of clairvoyant visions does not necessarily prevent the violent brain from engendering a precrime-like system—that is, treating the susceptible individual as soon-to-be criminal.

THE PROMISE OF THE VIOLENT BRAIN

There are several overlapping lines of thought concerning the therapeutic function of the violent brain model. Interestingly, a common intervention is to use this knowledge to advocate improvement in diet or lived environments. Along with such "social" interventions, neuroscientists also hope that by using this model they can identify susceptible individuals in at-risk populations and help them ward off antisocial tendencies. The goal here is to help such individuals realize and understand their neural shortcomings so that they may better manage their risk for violence. Relatedly, then, neuroscientists also propose that the violent brain model will pinpoint biomarkers that will help *predict* the risk for future offending, or recidivism. There are, however, conflicting ideas concerning the populations, communities, and/or behaviors that will be the target of the violent brain model.

Some interventions seem to imply that the violent brain model is a tool for any individual exhibiting violent and/or criminal behaviors. Others remain much closer to the program's mental health approach, limiting the technology to individuals with personality disorders. And some neuroscientists view the intervention capabilities of the violent brain much more liberally, making them applicable to *any* individual, violent or normal, as a way to elucidate the potential for neurobiological risk for violence. As it turns out, however, none of these groupings is mutually exclusive in practice. Interventions that focus on mental health disorders do not necessary exclude "normal" or "healthy" individuals who may one day be at risk. Nevertheless, all of these hypothetical uses for the neuroscience of violence are bound together by a particular vision of potentiality in the violent brain model.

The violent brain model does not function as a back door for neuroscientists to experiment and lobotomize away an individual's risks for violence. Today, the therapeutic function of the program is based on a tempered and discursive *therapeutic promise*—an embodiment of the practice of anticipation.[3] That is, the therapeutic promise is an imaginary whose epistemic value rests in the logic that "with each day [neuroscientists] can be closer to detecting abnormalities [for] useful interventions . . . [and] as technologies keep on improving, [neuroscientists], as clinicians, will keep on getting better too."[4] This promise operates by suspending the desire for an immediate cure for violence, replacing such a demand with a tentative potentiality to unlock curative secrets about violence for the future. Take the following comments from Dr. Lewis:

> The fantasy would be to cure psychopaths so that they're not a problem anymore, don't commit any crimes, and don't become serial killers. However, that might be a little ambitious in one lifetime. Just to contribute to a body of knowledge that might be more useful for future generations to study and work with would still be very valuable.[5]

Here, it is the openness of neurobiological knowledges for violence, its reflexive, if not uncertain, characteristic that neuroscientists draw upon to both rationalize their work and also seek to expand the areas to which to apply brain technologies of violence. Thus, neuroscientists are both working through the past to help quell old debates about the program and "constantly trying to understand the present by borrowing from a cautiously imagined emergent future, filled with volatility, and uncertainty."[6]

Starting with its making and continuing through its practice in the lab and anticipated application in society, the violent brain model actively demarcates who should use it and how, where (in society) it will be used, and upon which populations it will work best. The therapeutic promise constitutes and melds together, or coproduces, neuroscientific interpretations with societal realities; it is part of the larger discursive framework that helps convince others—the state, institutions, and possible patients—of its life-saving, -creating, and -altering potentials. These potentials become ever more tangible when thought about as different forms of capital in society: traditional *economic expenditures* (e.g., the violent brain model as a more efficient way to reduce violence, and therefore reduce financial cost), *cultural resources* (i.e., by identifying areas of the brain in need of improvement, the violent brain model may help individuals increase their own pro-social assets), and especially *promissory value* (i.e., the violent brain model offers boundless intervention possibilities).

Promissory value is not unique to the violent brain model, but commonplace in contemporary risk-thinking discourses of biomedicine.[7] It represents the malleability of new biotechnical systems of knowledge and life, and the idea that when employed properly such systems will continually create value in the form of potentialities.[8] Sociologist Charis Thompson uses the concept to capture the way reproductive technologies have refashioned the human embryo; now "constitutively promissory," its value "stems from its life creating potential."[9] Following Thompson, Beatrix Rubin traces the "therapeutic promise" that underlies embryonic stem cell research. Rubin points to the way scientific proposals—potential uses for and examinations of human stem cell research—transform how the human embryo is managed: reframing how it can be manipulated in the lab, debated in the public sphere, and regulated in the legal and policy realms.[10] The therapeutic promise is also meant to capture how the speculative intention of biotechnology is bound to its social practice. Such intersections, between imaginary and praxis, are flexible but also inextricable, such that the therapeutic promise helps bind the scientific function and social expectations of the violent brain model, while simultaneously helping to manage, if not obscure, the social and biopolitical complexities that threaten its existence and function. Therefore, though the therapeutic promise does not fully subdue the threats of social control, this discursive practice rewires its pathways, opening up new tracks toward biomedicalized surveillance *and* the re-production, if not further entrenchment, of social inequality through the emergence of a new kind of criminal, the *susceptible individual*.[11]

First conceptualized by Nikolas Rose, the susceptible individual is a "person with an elevated neurobiological risk of being the perpetrator of aggression or violence."[12] This new criminal is a product of "screen and intervene"—a manifestation of governmentality that emerged together with the promise of the brain sciences.[13] In practice, the susceptible individual overlaps and fluidly transverses several classifications attached to the violent brain model—"criminal," "pathological," and "normal." Therefore, the therapeutic promise is inseparable from the susceptible individual; each plays a vital role in the constitution of the other through an entwined lens of prediction *and* management.

Moreover, the key to the emergence of this new kind of criminal is not what the susceptible individual *is* at this moment, but what this potential criminal *can* be or *will* act like in the future. That is, this individual's predictive qualities, and not his or her ontological character, are what makes this category promising and useful for today's neuroscientists. The brain becomes the site of transformation, although always an unfinished one that is never fully capable of achieving the transformations needed to thwart violence. A cure per se, is not even an imagined goal; rather, the source of the promise is instead that new neuroscientific knowledge may help an individual to continually work on his or her brain in order to reduce the *risk* of violence. The efficacy of the therapeutic promise, then, depends on how well a neurobiological framing of violence can convince and instruct the susceptible individual to recognize the behavioral risk (ideals that are already uncertain and indeterminant) and manage behavioral tendencies.

"THERE ARE NO CURES"

As noted above, the therapeutic promise implies a hope for a future intervention, a commitment to the science as the best way to address violence in society. However, there is not agreement among neuroscientists about this promise. "I don't find that there's ever going to be a neurobiological explanation of violence," stated Dr. Lewis in our conversation.[14] While seemingly paradoxical, this comment actually makes sense when viewed through the lens of the therapeutic promise. An implicit distinction is being made here that can be traced directly to the "fitting" process, a symbolic parsing of the meaning of violence as destructive behavior in general and as a specific feature of clinical disorders like psychopathy or antisocial behavior. The former conceptualization is too uncertain and multifaceted for a neurobiological explanation—an implicit admission that not all violent behaviors are suitable for the violent brain model. Fitting, on the other hand, implies that a neurobiological explanation will pertain only to the clinical disorder; violence in this sense is a symptom of that disorder.

Other neuroscientists are more direct. They believe that neurobiology will provide needed answers about the etiology of mental disorders, but they do not expect that such knowledges will produce a cure. "The more we characterize violent behavior in terms of its neurobiological and genetic underpinnings, and the social underpinnings in those interactions, the more people will see that it's not simple,"[15] Dr. Jones tells me while discussing the prospect of a cure for violence. Then Dr. Jones flatly stated:

> You know—all these words like "cure" and "deterministic," they don't exist. Even in medicine, *there are no cures.* . . . You have a headache, you take Advil. It doesn't cure your headache. It just manages some symptoms. If you have an underlying problem the headache will come back. So the medical system is geared around *minimizing* symptoms. . . . But people will still say, "cure, cure, cure," you know. I get letters from people in jail that saw the program or heard about me, asking "Can I be cured?" It's very sad, but—there is no cure. [16]

From Dr. Jones's comments we can see that there remains an ardent sense of trust in the power of neurobiology to provide some useful information about violence. However, for Dr. Jones the violent brain model is not (and will not be) a panacea. The theoretical promise, then, is not premised on the eradication of violence from society, but on an anticipation that greater knowledge and technoscientific practices can pinpoint the molecular source of bad behavior and produce interventions that can effectively *minimize* the symptoms that arise from such risk.

"Minimizing symptoms" strengthens the medical model of violence, even as it suggests a more realistic outcome—that the underlying problem, certain personality disorders, remains elusive or outside the reach of a cure. At its best, the violent brain may be able to offer treatment options to help individuals learn how to cope with their violent symptoms or neuropsychological urges—emotional or cognitive decision-making abilities—that may increase the tendency for antisocial traits or behaviors. This is what embodies the violent brain's creative potential, what drives the anticipation that the violent brain is the unheralded "solution" to societal problems with violence. That is, even without a "cure" it will provide patently indispensable knowledge that will help individuals live with their mental illness and, in the eyes of proponents, move society closer to a complete understanding of what makes a person behave violently.

It is worth noting that researchers may *already* be overselling the therapeutic potential of the violent brain. As noted above, one public audience (incarcerated populations) is being persuaded by its possible healing abilities more than by neuroscientists themselves. This becomes a tricky situation for neuroscientists to navigate, to subdue the current therapeutic expectations of the violent brain, while also promoting its importance as a medical disorder, and a potentially more complete answer for violence in society. Another neuroscientist I spoke with noted that some incarcerated or violent populations feel more empowered to rebuff the stigmatization of mental illness if there is neurobiological proof of brain disease. Such individuals "feel better hearing that there's a real [medical] problem [causing their behavior]; because they're not crazy if they have a condition that other people have."[17] Dumit describes this phenomenon as a refashioning of the "objective-self."[18] Through neurobiological models of mental illness, the "objective-self" provides a space to discover, remake, and manage personhood. The seemingly resolute boundaries of defining the criminal no longer hold sway, and the person instead reshapes his or her identity through a medical explanation of deviancy, in which a new biomedical identity is realized. "The relations between the two selves are redistributed so that although the patient must continue to experience the illness and live with it, she or he no longer has to identify with it. The diseased brain, in this case, becomes a part of a biological body that is experienced phenomenologically but is not the bearer of personhood."[19] Thus, where the patient sees an infallible medical explanation, a more humanizing and sympathetic identity versus that of a criminal, the neuroscientist perceives an "object" of science.

For the neuroscientist, uncovering the neurobiological makeup of a susceptible individual specifies a person perpetually at risk and unable to be cured, but potentially manageable with the right diagnosis and treatment.

It is not clear if such populations come to conceptualize violent behavior as a legitimate medical problem or as a symptom of a psychological disorder, but the therapeutic promise seems to rationalize this medicalized interpretation of violence as a result of one's inability of choice. Adding to this delicate dilemma, many suggested that neurobiological treatments for the violence are not exclusively "medical" in any manner. In fact, most of these interventions for minimizing the risk for violence seem to be very similar to the "social" prevention policies proposed by social scientists and public health officials.[20]

PREVENTION AS CHANGING BRAINS

Raine has long emphasized the need for better childhood nutrition and environmental enrichment as ways to combat the risk for violence.[21] Broadly speaking, chronic childhood hunger has been linked to an increased vulnerability for adverse health effects later in life.[22] In terms of violent behavior, at least two studies have found a decrease in antisocial behavior for individuals placed on diets rich in omega-3s,[23] although subsequent work and reviews of this intervention have been mixed.[24] A study conducted at a Dutch prison found that prisoners given daily supplements (vitamins, antioxidants, and minerals) demonstrated a 34 percent reduction in reported aggressive or rule-breaking incidents compared to prisoners taking placebo supplements.[25] However, the authors found no significant changes in psychological function for individuals in the study, meaning that there was no clear indication that prisoners' behavioral changes were due to antecedent changes in neurobiological or neuropsychological function, or that such changes in fact blunted more-serious behaviors like violence. The lack of correlation among nutritional intake, behavior, and the brain, however, does not necessarily undercut claims that diet affects behavior. It does, though, complicate—if not disrupt— the causal associations made about mental disorders, diet, and behavior.

This study did not distinguish prisoners with clinical disorders from those without a diagnosis, but the design "shortcoming" nevertheless seems to support the idea that nutritional supplements may have some impact on social behavior, more broadly speaking. Further, the authors also noted that the link between poor diet and behavior may be limited by age, in which there may be a "critical window" of time when such an intervention will have the most benefit. Age also restricts the benefits of this intervention for violence, which has pushed neuroscientists to think more seriously about critical periods of intervention.

Critical windows of development focus on the "early identification of people who are on a 'life-course persistent' pathway, [with the goal] to help better optimize their treatment, or help ensure that [they] get off the life-course pathway as a way to reduce their risk of going to criminal courts or prisons in adulthood."[26] Life-course-persistent individuals are thought to represent a small subset of the population that engages in antisocial acts at a young age and continues throughout adulthood.[27] However, "life-course-persistent individual" is not a unique biomedical classification. The population represents a more general criminological taxonomy, and some researchers believe that the group may make up a larger proportion of offenders with criminal convictions.

Sociologists have also been interested in life-course models; however, some of them have criticized biological understandings of these developmental trajectories because they often designate social dynamics as immutable empirical objects. Sociologist Robert Sampson and criminologist John Laub write that "while most developmentalists allude to social interactions as real, in the end most embrace a focus that emphasizes the primacy of early childhood attributes that are presumed to be stable over the life course in a between-individual sense."[28] Their critique calls into question how well neurobiological readings of life course can handle social variability—that is, ongoing variations in social environments, life choices, and presumably even biosocial conditioning. Moreover, this question is brought into even sharper focus through neurobiological interventions that focus on environmental enrichment from the Mauritius Child Health Project.[29]

Although the interventions in the project were limited to participants in the study, they were compelling examples of the necessity of social approaches to health and behavior. The project proposed "the promotion of better socialization of the child, the encouragement of imaginative and creative play to foster cognitive development . . . and a structured daily schedule with varied activities."[30] This manifested as practical social strategies that the neuroscientists used as research measures: the building of a nursery school and training for teachers, health screening and physical exercise, home visits and counseling for parents and students, and a nutritional program that provided lunch. Such approaches are similar to the more holistic violence-prevention strategies pushed for by health experts in the United States.[31] Thus, we see that neuroscientists and social scientists do not always differ in terms of the types of interventions recommended to help reduce violence (in general).

Clearly we cannot, and should not, turn neighborhoods into lab sites as a means of generating safer communities. However, neuroscientific suggestions for socially based interventions for violence represent an interesting, and thorny, test for critics. If the power of the violent brain can better convince societies (and particularly policy-makers) of the effectiveness of social interventions to prevent violence, then should social scientists also leverage this technology to help secure needed social resources and attention to violence in our society? One looming concern here is the way neuroscientists conceptualize the significance of social interventions. Some neuroscientists narrowly interpret the importance of social interventions, like nutritional intake, as a way to *change* the brain.

Applying an understanding of change that is akin to the notion of *neuroplasticity*—the belief that the brain is always "becoming" but never fixed[32]—neuroscientists hope that social-based intervention will help individuals develop healthier brains during these critical periods of development. Neurobiological knowledges of violence shape, and reshape, the underlying purpose and effectiveness of existing social interventions. Supplemental intake is reimagined as a means of blunting the effects of genetic predispositions that produce neurologic risk for antisocial behavior. Similarly, enhancing social relationships is thought to help cultivate "neurocognitive abilities" that are deemed fundamental for warding off unwanted behavioral traits. That is, food (nutritional intake), the environment, and social experiences are repacked through the violent brain model, as unique and calculable kinds of neurobiological *exposures* that help influence brain development and future brain functioning.[33] To be clear, I am not arguing against providing better diets or improved living conditions; instead I am questioning the definitional and practical ways that the violent brain, once again, casually blurs the line between violence as a neurobiological marker and more-general causes of violence in society.[34] Even as the violent brain endorses interventions at the sociocultural level, it is also restricting—or more specifically, individualizing—their importance to the brain as the optimal location to properly detect and assess preventive impacts.

NEUROBIOLOGICAL RESPONSIBILITY

One of the most difficult populations to treat is children with callous-unemotional (CU) traits. Remember that CU is essentially a designation for youth with psychopathic traits. Similar to psychopathy, genetic factors are thought to influence CU, yet neuroscientists make clear that the true risk for violence in this population is primarily driven by environmental experiences that may act upon and through such neurobiological factors.[35] As mentioned before, genetic risk for violence is inseparable from environmental context, but what is reiterated here is that despite the focus on neurobiological makeup during diagnosis, environmental exposures may matter more for prevention and treatment. Neuroscientists Essi Viding and Eamon McCory, leading experts on callous-unemotional (CU) traits, reject the idea that biomedical interventions like gene therapy, the experimental technique that alters genetic makeup to correct harmful genetic mutations thought to cause "untreatable" diseases, may work as a treatment for CU.[36] They instead posit that the most effective interventions for CU are based on improving the sociocultural interactions between children and their parental guardians.[37] Similarly, other neuroscientists working with CU populations also recommend social-based interventions that "work with parents and the child to try and make sure that they're rewarding good behaviors, and that they're being structured and predictable in the way they punish bad behaviors."[38] The violent brain, then, is not only constructing the bounds of the optimal susceptible individual—in this case children or *susceptible children*—but also anticipating a new kind of parenting.

There is a self-disciplining property at the intersection of neuroplasticity and the violent brain, which reminds us that the susceptible individual is constantly in formation, always being worked upon, never fully complete. What seems to separate the susceptible individual from the criminal in general is not simply a clinical diagnosis, but a fundamental belief—a not-so-subtle expectation—that the susceptible individual will minimize and work upon his or her own neurobiological (in)abilities by actively seeking the right social environments to cultivate, if not accelerate, brain plasticity. This version of responsibility expands the same requirement to the parents or families of the susceptible individual. Carlos Novas and Nikolas Rose noted that genetic responsibility "intersects with, and becomes allied to, contemporary norms of selfhood that stress autonomy, self-actualization, prudence, responsibility and choice."[39] Unlike in some situations of genetic responsivity, parents here are not being blamed, or blaming themselves, for their child's inheritance of neurobiological riskiness for violence.[40] Here, neurobiological responsibility works as a type of agreement between parents and clinicians. The parents or guardians of a susceptible child are asked to both understand and supply the right type of environmental settings and educate their children about the wrong type of exposures so that their children—more specifically, their children's brains—can mitigate, and potentially eliminate, risks for violence.

The first step for parents or families is early recognition of the clinical signs or symptoms that may encourage antisocial behaviors. While explaining the potential to treat individuals diagnosed with antisocial behavior disorder during our interview, Dr. Moore details a description of conduct disorder, and the importance of early detection, which helps contextualize the reasoning behind neurobiological responsibility. "For people [with] conduct disorder, you know you're impulsive, you may be damaging property, you may be ill-treating animals—[overall] it is quite apparent that the person has a lot of behavioral symptoms. You feel out of control with siblings in the home environment or perhaps even in the school environment. It can lead to truancy and lower education attainment, and often a life of crime. So, if you really want to go back to what contributes to this disorder. So yeah, you can say that [antisocial disorders] possibly start from childhood—rather than somebody developing the disorder overnight in their adult years"[41] Neuroscientists, however, are not just seeking help from parents to recognize these factors during childhood. They are also implying that parents act upon these signs of risk.

Parental accountability, in this sense, suggests that parents have a responsibility to develop the right kinds of brains in children, ostensibly "normal" or "healthy" brains, able to counteract neurobiological risks. Children's brains, then, can be understood as a form of "cerebral architecture," an ambitious prototype through which "good self-governance" can be developed or sculpted with the right kind of parenting.[42] Neuroscientific understandings about the development of healthy brains, and their implied ability as a natural buffer for risk, are inseparable from societal conceptions of maturity—i.e., a fully developed or properly developed brain is a healthy and normal one, ostensibly free of risk factors for violence. However, this reinterpretation of social mechanisms as neurobiological fixes can take for granted the stratified and uneven distribution of social resources in society.

Socioeconomic factors, like employment, income, and wealth, may limit the ability of families to provide certain social resources that are vital for brain development. Sociologist Victoria Pitts-Taylor makes a similar argument regarding the neuroscience of poverty, in which changing brains is also seen as the optimal strategy to combat the effects of poverty among young children. Like violence, the many impacts of poverty are varied, and often more social and political in nature than biological. The purpose of this critique is not to dismiss the idea that childhood poverty may manifest as embodied biosocial effects. Instead, it highlights how neuroscientific interventions can constrain biosocial dynamics to specific, and often contradictory, configurations that actually "fix" certain persons (brains) to existing social arrangements of social power in order to understand their neurobiological import.[43]

Likewise, research from Kasia Tolwinski shows that "plasticity-talk" has been used as a rebuttal to criticism, particularly scientific racism, that has been leveled at this theory of "broken brains."[44] Although these neuroscientists certainly recognize, and hope, that their work addresses social inequality, Tolwinski finds that their attempts to manage controversy using less-determinist claims, or even projected personal social justice leanings, have not led to an amelioration, at least not in the bioethical sense, of the science as thought. Instead, neuroscientists who have revived historically troublesome areas of biological research, like poverty or violence, via neurobiological methods are continually operating in what Tolwinski calls a "fraught research terrain." Pitts-Taylor's and Tolwinski's findings remind us that neuroscientists who present neuroplasticity as a solution to social problems without taking existing power dynamics seriously are inviting systemic inequalities to be reconstituted through their work, since "the measurement of human difference through biosocial plasticity can require cuts that belie biosocial complexity and that (mis)construe the experience of individuals and groups as homogenous and predictable."[45] The focus on developing healthy young brains is as much a sociocultural notion as it is a scientific fact, and the responsibility may subject parents and families from marginalized communities who are unable to completely fulfill their roles to disproportionately higher levels of scrutiny.

Dorothy Roberts makes clear that there is a politic undergirding the criminalization of parenting that has been used to target poor African American mothers through state sanction threats to their reproductive and guardianship rights.[46] In this way, neurobiological responsibility may go beyond helping neuroscientists find a way to minimize the risk for violence. Instead, the obligation may unwittingly link social understandings of "poor parenting" to future violence. That is, "poor parenting" may act as a neurobiological proxy to help *predict* susceptible individuals.[47] Charlotte Walsh notes that the belief that "poor parenting" is the primary cause of violent children is still embedded within social policies in the United States and the United Kingdom, and that such ideologies have preserved the right of the state to intervene, or even dictate, parenting decisions for families as a means of preventing crime.[48] Parenting alone is not the only measure used to predict violence, but it does highlight another interesting characteristic of the violent brain, *neuroprediction* as an intervention.

NEUROPREDICTION

From its first conceptualization, the violent brain model was built to predict, to provide some knowledge about one's chances of being violent. Prediction, in the general sense, suggests an ability to see into the future. In the neurosciences, prediction refers to the statistical meaning of the term—more like an average, or optimal, outcome, given the variables used in a model.[49] This type of predictive power is why neuroscientists invest in the violent brain. Risk calculations can never be as precise or specific as neuroscientists would like; as Dr. McKinney told me, "It's like asking the weatherman to predict who's going to get struck by lightning. I can give you some percentages, but no, I can't tell you who's going to get struck by lightning."[50]

This is also why neuroscientists comfortably argued that the violent brain is not determinist, because it works in terms of probabilities. "I think that there's an agreement, really an agreement among scientists that violence is multifactorial," another neuroscientist replied. "It's really complex and cannot be predicted one hundred percent and not even ninety percent, and that is something that all of the scientists you interview will agree with."[51] The commitment to prediction, then, has much more to do with the ability to better elucidate important group-level and clinical details about personality disorders associated with violent behavior. Although neuroscientists are not promising to predict violent behavior with certainty, the use of neuroimaging tools rests on a promise to help "decode what an individual is thinking from their brain activity."[52]

Neuroprediction, or "brain-reading," as it is sometimes called, is an ultimate goal of neuroimaging research,[53] but it also takes on a greater importance for the study of violence. The violent brain's perceived ability to read one's future through brain structure and function cultivates hope and promise not just as a research tool, but also as a potential treatment for otherwise incurable abnormal social behaviors. Prediction operates on multiple levels through the violent brain. First, neuroimaging is used to outline and determine neurobiological biomarkers (an overactive amygdala, or a smaller prefrontal cortex). Next, using group-level analyses (average differences between clinical and control groups), the (dys)function of such biomarkers is linked to neuropsychological diagnosis. Finally, these bio-markers are further targeted in the development of interventions, often social practices that are thought to help minimize or correct the impact of these risk factors on brain functioning. Yet this logic carries salient shortcomings, especially when considering the burgeoning relationship between neuroscience and the law.

The use of neuroscience in the law is not new, as this book has highlighted with several examples of the use of neurotechnologies in the courtroom. Since the mid-2000s, there has been an urgent uptake of neuroscience in the realm of law. Some scholars within the subfield of neurolaw have advocated a greater use of neuroscientific discoveries to advance legal and social policy.[54] However, attorneys have also sought to introduce neurobiological knowledges as evidence in the courtroom. According to legal and ethics scholars Henry Greely and Nita Farahany, defenses based on neurobiological evidence—what they characterize as the "their brains made them do it"—were introduced in nearly 2,800 judicial opinions in the United States between 2005 and 2015.[55]

In the 2005 Supreme Court case *Roper v. Simmons*, the Court relied upon neuroscientific findings on brain maturity in its ruling that outlawed the death penalty for adolescents (people 18 or younger). It is common to perceive adolescence as a developing age, in which people do not understand fully the consequences of their actions. However, *Roper v. Simmons* also demonstrates how social ideologies can be taken up into scientific practices without question, and further harden. Adolescents, as a social group, are as multifarious and flexible as the socially constructed meanings for "violent offenders" or "criminals." Neuroscientists are not necessarily challenging these meanings, but they are uncritically accepting them as exact and demonstrable measures in their work. Moreover, as Dumit points out, there are links here, not just one between age and maturity but also a more intricate one between maturity and "dangerousness."[56]

Neuroscientists' attempt to link the narratives of maturity and dangerousness makes more sense if we think about the underlying neurobiological description of violence as a clinical inability to regulate one's emotions or control decision making. However, such brain understandings seem less convincing when the individual is a "mature" adult, with a fully developed brain. This is not to say that neuroscientists' findings are fabrications, but that measurable differences are as much about our social understandings with regard to maturity, dangerousness, and development as they are scientific proof of brain function and shape.[57] Moreover, the role of neuroscience in the courts has expanded well beyond its original evidentiary function.

Neuro-knowledges are thought to provide more-informative and -objective truths regarding philosophical debates about legal responsibility, and fMRI scans have been touted as the future of lie detectors and powerful devices to uncover hidden implicit biases among jurors, judges, and attorneys.[58] The expansive application of these neurotechnologies in the courtroom will only increase the chance that such knowledges may be misused, or used beyond their functional limit through the law. Neuroscientists and other legal experts have attempted to educate legal professionals about the way neuroscience should and should not be used in the courtroom to help reduce this risk. The point is well illustrated in a publication from the MacArthur Foundation Research Network on Law and Neuroscience at Vanderbilt University. The stated purpose of *A Judges' Guide to Neuroscience* is to address questions and concerns that judges, lawyers, and other legal experts may have about the role of neuroscience in the courtroom. However, such attempts to demystify neuroscience may expand the authority for the violent brain. Interviewee Dr. McKinney has worked with judges and other legal professionals. McKinney's comments also suggest that the training of judges will help the legal world to better grasp the importance of neuroscience data. However, as Dr. McKinney contended:

I've discovered that the only way to really make a change is not to convince through behavioral and clinical evidence, even though I honestly and fundamentally believe it is *much* more informative and better, but we are going to have to show [judges] pictures of brains.[59]

The argument here is not atypical. As noted in Chapter 3, the colorful display of the brain carries its own authority, which may do a far better job at convincing lay audiences of the importance of the violent brain than less-accessible statistical equations or charts. This type of "neuro-training" in the courtroom also has consequences. Neuroscientists rely on judges, as judicial gatekeepers, to ensure that understandings of the violent brain will be properly applied in the courts. However, preparing judges to know *how* to "see" the violent brain works against neuroscientists' stated goals, as it entices judges to believe in the powers of brain imaging without fully understanding its predictive powers and especially its scientific shortcomings. This increases the chances that such visualizations are accepted as evidence that seemingly speaks for itself.[60]

These hurdles for translating neuroscience knowledge are not limited to misinterpretations of brain scans. A fundamental problem with prediction through the violent model is the lack of power in predictive models. This has led some neuroscientists studying violence to reject the use of certain biomarkers for violence in the courtroom, as Dr. Fitzpatrick told me:

There were a couple years in which we would regularly be called by people who were interested in using [our research] as evidence in death penalty hearings, or [asking] if someone has the MAOA low variant, does that mean it should be taken into account [during such a hearing]— whether or not they should receive the death penalty. My own position is that [the research] is not material because the risk increase from MAOA is so minor that it would do very little towards explaining or exculpating individual violent acts, no matter how heinous. So, I'm not in favor of that kind of approach.[61]

While this comment focuses on the role of the MAOA variant, it underscores the fact that neuroscientists did not construct the violent brain with the goal of adjudicating an individual's innocence or guilt of a crime in the legal sphere. Like MAOA, other neurobiological biomarkers also yield small effect sizes, and therefore may not bring about the dramatic adjudicative or therapeutic impact expected from scientific technologies. That is, they explain only a very small amount of the variance, and therefore cannot account for other effects, sociocultural or biological, that may be in play during the act of violence. Moreover, Dr. Fitzpatrick's comments illuminate the "group-to-individual" (G2i) problem. As noted in Chapter 3, the point of neuroscience research is to provide a more general picture of violence, and therefore findings represent group averages. "Pictures" of violent, moral, or normal brains are representations that obscure individual variability. Simply comparing individuals' brain scans using these representations of the "antisocial brain," therefore, cannot prove anything particular about that individual's past behavior; again, brain scans are not intended to diagnose.

Other neuroscientists, however, have tried to better circumscribe the role of prediction for the criminal justice system. Kiehl's mobile MRI lab intends to predict the likelihood of rearrests or reoffending, focusing on future criminality and ostensibly operating outside the realm of culpability. In one study, Kiehl and colleagues successfully linked neural activation in the anterior cingulate cortex (ACC) region of the brain, an area associated with conflict monitoring, with felony arrest.[62] The group noted that the use of the violent brain here may provide some predictive advantage over existing behavioral models of risk assessment, which are already used in parole decisions. In this sense, the violent brain is supposed to be used alongside these existing risk assessments to provide more-accurate risk estimates.[63] However, there remain ethical questions about using the brain to predict recidivism. Recidivism is not just an indication of criminal behavior (violent or nonviolent), but like any other arrest, it also reflects sociocultural dynamics that help dictate where, when, and upon whom to police. Kiehl's group actually acknowledged this dynamic themselves in their latest publication:

> It is important to recognize that accuracy equally applies to the outcome variables as it does the predictor variables. Here we have used official arrest reports to derive our primary outcome variable (re-arrest), such reports may be biased by police strategies, geography, profiling, etc. Future studies may consider using both self-report data on criminal activities as well as arrest reports to assess whether one may be more accurate than another.[64]

This admission is noteworthy, as it demonstrates a better recognition of the multifactorial nature of violence, and the way social power influences the way society thinks about and responds to violence. However, predicting violence is a comprehensive political social practice, symbiotically indebted to the types of policing practices employed in communities.

Scholars have shrewdly noted that the landscapes of criminal justice and social geographies, and the reporting and tracking practices that are used to enable and sustain these systems, are heavily implicated in American society's systematic reproduction of racial, class, and gendered inequities.[65] Therefore, noting that biased policing strategies could have skewed a primary outcome variable, but still relying on these data to provide some neutral neurobiological narrative about recidivism, undermines the critical admission expressed in the article. The concern here is not about accuracy or a more accurate account of arrests (either merely provides a quantitative data point, without taking into account problematic social dynamics). Here again, we see an interesting negation that is inherent to the violent brain construct. On the one hand, embedded practices of inequality are admittingly rendered too complex for this model (as shown in Chapter 5). However, and on the other hand, the very same complexity, here in the form of policing records, is nevertheless rendered workable and relied upon as a vital research variable, when codified through scientific practices of the brain.

Dr. Holmes, another neuroscientist who encourages the use of neuroprediction, envisions a slightly different role for the violent brain in terms of preventing recidivism. The outlined goal for Dr. Holmes is to better address long-sought answers concerning why some individuals continue to commit crimes or behave violently, while others do not, an intervention that could help elucidate both the neurobiology of violence and *resilience*. Here, the renewed therapeutic promise of the violent brain is more explicitly tied to violence-prevention programs, to "test the efficacy of community intervention programs in the scanner." Dr. Holmes explains that

> the experiment would place at-risk youth in the scanner and have them do various sorts of decision-making tasks with and without somebody watching them over on a video feed. The youth would know they're being watched, and that they're being watched either by a peer or by a community elder; we already know that behaviorally, people will behave different

under those circumstances. So then, the question is, "Neurally, why do they behave differently in those circumstances?" Now, that may or may not be useful information. The way it could be useful is if we discover that "You know what? People's behavior really changes when—I'll just make something up—the dorsolateral prefrontal cortex comes online because they're being watched by someone they respect." In theory, we could test the efficacy of several different community intervention programs in the scanner—in other words, we can say, "Alright, well what would it be like, if instead of having a former gang member watching them, we have their grandmother watch them? What would it be like if we have a police officer watch them? What would it be like if we have their school principal watch them?" We could compare the efficacy of different community intervention programs, not by having to run them in the community one at a time, but instead by understanding the associated neural signatures—like thinking ahead and not acting with reactive violence—from these youth.[66]

Dr. Holmes's vision would also be revolutionary for violence prevention. If successful, it could demonstrate the value of preventive strategies for violence, which often do not yield immediate results and require substantial economic investment, community trust, and political buy-in. However, it also suggests that the violent brain model can cleanse data of its social, and potentially unequal, nature. There's a theoretical leap made here between social perception and actual social behavior—that potential behavior outside the lab can be known based on recorded differences in brain activity when social peers or guardians watch the participant. It is accurate to think that individuals may behave differently when they are with different social groups, but this seems to suggest that youth will behave violently only in front of their peers, and that they will always behave properly in the presence of guardians or authoritative adults. Given that participating in such a study requires a willingness from at-risk youth to abide by the rather stringent guidelines for imaging and for them to be observed within a lab, it is unlikely that they will behave differently, or inappropriately, when they believe a peer is watching them. It is also unlikely that a lab experiment can replicate social environments or experiences that would lead to antisocial behavior. What this means is that this intervention takes for granted the interrelationships between social actions and social terrain, which are vital to explanations of violence or its risk factors.

Maybe the most difficult barrier for neuroprediction will be the public. Even with these sophisticated statistical and technological interpretations of neuroprediction, neuroscientists will still need to convince the public that the violent brain's public good will outweigh its perceived risk. Risk in this sense is not simply a question of stigmatization due to biomedical labels like antisocial or psychopathy, which nearly all the neuroscientists I talked with noted as a potential social concern, but societal-level fears of deterministic-like regimes of prediction. By now, it should be clear that when neuroscientists say a person is at risk for violence it does not mean a destiny for crime. However, such reassurances have not completely shut the door on deterministic thinking, either.

"MINORITY REPORT" (AGAIN)

I started this chapter with a brief discussion of "Minority Report." This vision is "revived" in a speculative work of fiction by Raine. In this neurobiological vision of precrime, Legal Offensive on Murder: Brain Research Operation for Screening of Offenders, or the acronym LOMBROSO, a long-term surveillance and detention idea underscores the actual fears and concerns that critics of the neuroscience of violence voice today. Although Raine's story is fictitious, he does present a notice that the less-sophisticated precrime-like trends already exist. Thus, it presents a case for neurobiological knowledges of violence becoming a normal part of everyday life (if that has not already happened), to replace or improve upon existing crude operations of crime prediction in a more socially productive and ethically prudent manner.

In this future, LOMBROSO would require all "males" (again, the Y chromosome as a marker of maleness, and therefore aggression, is thought to be the most obvious, natural predictor of violence) to submit to a genetic screening and neuroimaging scan by the age of eighteen, the time when the brain is thought to be "mature." Those individuals who are found biologically risky for violent behaviors would be held indefinitely at designated detention centers, although not fully stripped of their citizenship rights (e.g., they can still vote).[67] Subsequent renditions of LOMBROSO, Raine muses, would include mandatory comprehensive screening for all children by age ten. Moreover, he considers the potential implementation of a "parenting license"—a type of governmental authorization that would help to ensure that individuals have the parenting skills needed to have a child, as "poor parenting" is portrayed as a key reason that a child may develop an unhealthy brain.

Raine seems to take a middle-ground approach toward a real-world version of his LOMBROSO prophecy.[68] He correctly warns of the real-world possibility that LOMBROSO is not too far-fetched, or as he put it, "the essence of the LOMBROSO program has been essentially alive and well for years in countries like England."[69] As an example, he points to the imprisonment for public protection (IPP) sentence in the UK, which allowed the police to arrest and detain any individual for a period of time under the vague reasoning of "public protection." This policy was in effect for seven years before being overturned in 2012. Yet the very fact that it was debated and enacted as a solution for crime should give us all pause about the realistic implementation of biologically based screening programs, or at the very least seamlessly interjecting neurobiological measures into such "precrime-like" models to make such policies seem more neutral, scientific, and necessary. The continuing expansion of criminal DNA databanks exemplifies this point well.

In both the United Kingdom and the United States the practice of familial DNA matching has been increasing.[70] The technique made national headlines in 2018 in the United States when it was used to apprehend Joseph James DeAngelo, known as the "Golden State Killer."[71] DeAngelo was arrested after a police search of the public DNA database *GEDmatch* found a match to his third-degree cousin.[72] Legal scholars have warned that such practices seem to allow law enforcement to sidestep privacy and constitutional concerns simply because of one's relationship to others who have been arrested or convicted.[73] The question here is not *if* such practices work—scientifically, these procedures can produce matches—but *how* they work. In the United States and the United Kingdom, where social inequities are inextricably bound to the way the criminal justice system functions, profiles that have already been collected will also illustrate such unequal sociopolitical practices. Therefore, when matches work, they may help to sustain, or make more efficient, an already problematic policing system.[74] The ability to question riskiness, and seemingly to evidence guilt, through familiar biological makeup should trigger larger, more fundamental social and ethical questions about privacy, ownership, and access to biometric data. Moreover, such concerns are not limited to the issue of violence.

In education, advocates of *sociogenomics* have recently pushed to use genetic markers of risk as the best chance to help close the academic achievement gap.[75] Similarly, there is a growing debate about immigration, as officials in both the United States and Europe are employing genetic technologies as a way to help reunite families separated at border checkpoints. Scholars have warned that such policies will institute an inherent social risk, that such genetics practices operate as a political tool that actually further separates, racializes, and *criminalizes* certain "fraudulent" immigrant families.[76] Importantly, such practices demonstrate the ever vanishing boundary that neuroscientists try to preserve between susceptible individuals and convicted or "known" violent subjects. Regimes of risk rarely need to distinguish between such labels, as societies, through existing mechanisms of power and ideologies of difference, tend to treat them all as "would-be-criminals"— always already potential threats to society.

Raine, while acknowledging concerns for programs like LOMBROSO, nevertheless notes that "the harsh reality of life is that we have to balance risk with benefits."[77] He goes on to describe a more optimistic function for LOMBROSO, one that centers on neurobiology as the missing piece for achieving effective violence interventions. Raine is not alone in this regard; most neuroscientists admit that the ethical and social challenges that accompany any intervention from neurobiological research on violence are counterbalanced by the future benefits of the science. However, these hopes for the violent brain construct are not definite; they are technoscientific *promises*—best-case scenarios that at once help researchers ease their own practical ambivalences to neuroprediction and thwart outside ethical challenges to the violent brain. While this promise makes it seem that the violent brain model has inherent and inevitable therapeutic capabilities, it does little to quell concerns about the preemptive use of coercive state power such as involuntary detention and confinement. Thus, pressing questions remain unanswered about the violent brain.

Who will and will not have access to such knowledges about violence both during and after they move beyond the lab? Here, privacy protections may collide with public welfare and safety policies that can make public one's past and potential criminal tendencies (e.g., the routine use of questions about criminal past on employment applications or efforts to expand public access to ex-felon registries).[78] Beyond privacy concerns, the already faint line that neuroscientists try to draw between "normal" and "risky" will be further blurred, if not completely erased, when the violent brain becomes evidentiary material for attorneys in the courtroom, a forensic device for police officers, a diagnostic instrument for health care providers, and/or a behavioral assessment tool for educators in the classroom. Any advantage gained through screenings for risk, then, could be offset by the threat of technological governance through this indiscriminate "regime of normativity."[79] Thus, interrogating the social consequences of this logic requires recognition of the existing and systemic forms of inequality that will dictate which individuals (or individual brains) will be viewed as being capable of change. The expectation for managing the neurobiological risk for violence will also be stratified along existing lines of social ideology and inequity. In other words, the susceptible individual is made, and refashioned, through the forces of power, inequality, and difference that neuroscientists have strategically avoided up to this point.

7 | THE LIMITS OF
SCIENTIFIC CONVICTION

THE VIOLENT BRAIN framework was born, and thrives, through controversy. It is the product of a contentious history, one that never really delivered the transformative knowledge about violence that was promised to the public and to the scientific world. Put differently, the violent brain represents the latest rendition of "failed science"—"poorly done, overinterpreted or biased" scientific ideas that have been discredited but nevertheless survived long after rejection.[1] Yet, if it is a "failure," it is an intriguing one.

Critics of the biology of violence will still stress the need for a more vociferous response from scientists themselves, for the makers of this knowledge to better educate the public about the ways in which flawed scientific knowledges lend support to dangerous social ideas. They will argue that scientific responsibility should compel neuroscientists to actively push back against misunderstandings and abuses of the knowledges that they produce. I agree with such pleas. Yet neuroscientists are not necessarily reproducing the same "flawed" ideas or arguments about biology and violence as in the past.

Conceptualizations of the violent brain have their limitations, as outlined throughout this book, but unlike the past attempts, such ideas are not easily reduced to descriptions like "junk science" or "pseudoscience." Nor are they, to invoke a standard sociological critique of the biosciences, straightforwardly "deterministic." Neuroscientists studying violence are respected researchers in the field, and their scientific methods differ very little from those of their contemporaries in the social and cognitive neurosciences. That is, contemporary models of the violent brain are built through the same neuroscientific and social psychological methods as are models of the social brain. This raises an interesting question for critics: what does a critique of the neuroscience of violence—as a potential despotic and social controlling force—say about social neuroscience research in general, and in particular the belief that democratic or liberating potentials lie within these new neuro-knowledges? So the critique here requires a bit more digging, to push past, or further interrogate what is really meant, or practiced, when neuroscience invokes the social as a defense against criticism

Violence, now "fitted" into a biomedical framework, becomes a symptom of neuropsychological disorder. Fitting engenders both a tangible technical practice and an ongoing discursive space of modification. Such practices displace the meaning of violent behavior from its legal or sociocultural framework and translate it into biomedical language. Fitting has, in a predictable fashion, stretched the promissory value of this model well beyond the bounds of clinical populations. The theoretical distinctions made between clinical groups and general criminal ones have never been as precise as neuroscientists suggest, and quite aptly, the violent brain logic collapses these categorical group distinctions with little resistance. Recognized by some neuroscientists, the blurring of distinctions between general violence and clinical disorders seems to threaten the value of the model and its predictive qualities. Neuroscientists have also utilized this empirical space to interpret, and reinterpret, the meanings of those "pictures" of antisocial, psychopathic, or criminal brains.

There has also been a renewed commitment to the social, actualized through the violent brain construct. These neuroscientific approaches to the social have been helpful in thwarting charges of determinism, but the real work seems to lie in examining how they are leveraged to suggest a sliding scale of brainhood. Essentially, social and antisocial individuals, according to this model, are polar opposites, the two ends of a continuum. At the "social" end, the brain is thought to work properly, without complications, or *normally;* at the other, antisocial end, the brain is presumably broken, workable in most social situations but constantly in need of better connections to achieve its optimal, risk-averting function. The empirical power of the violent brain, then, rests on a perceived ability to demonstrate where a group, or an individual, lies on this scale; to elucidate, and hopefully avert, the risk that one's brain may venture too close to the antisocial extreme. However, neuroscientists rarely explain *how* the violent brain model's instinctive bioethical stance works. Also, it remains unclear how a biosocial brain, beyond quantifying social/environmental factors, helps to naturally facilitate a socially responsible science.

If this is a failed science, its failures arise from its inability to recognize the limits of the scientific method, not from a simple lack of ethical sympathy or social acumen. Close attention to the way neuroscientists assemble and enact the violent brain model illuminates, and foreshadows, the unnoticed technological gaps that limit the model's ability to deal with the social stickiness attached to violent behavior. The reason many social scientists and critics push back against biological understandings of violence, ostensibly opting for "nurture" *over* "nature," has less to do with winning the nature/nurture debate or being right. Instead, social scientists have recognized that biological theories of behavior lack the ability to deal with the complexity of "social facts." Now we understand that the violent brain model also fails in this respect. It seems that it is better to explore the potential connections between the brain and violence and "fail," than to remain in the dark about a potentially complete picture of violence.

THE FAILURE OF CONVICTION

Contemporary neuroscience has reimagined the brain as a vital pathway point through which the social must pass—the critical meeting space or "inescapable nexus where [dynamic social] forces meet [the biological]."[2] The use of this epistemic in the biology of violence, while both novel and crucial for survival of the research program, has been marred with incomplete conceptualizations and management of social and environmental forces. At times, neuroscientists are able to work with the social, developing promising neurobiological measures thought to be influenced by particular environmental exposures. Yet, in other instances they inexplicably ignore or constrain dynamic social experiences. Through the violent brain model, researchers continually rework and realign the precarious social-biological connections with violence, but they never quite fully explicate the unique meaning of the "inescapable nexus" for violent behavior.

Attempts to piece together a convincing, workable neurobiological picture of violence illuminate an *in*ability to truly handle sociocultural dynamics through a violent brain model. This framework is not simply exposing the bonds between the biological and the social; it is also reassembling them, refitting social-biological entanglements, engagements, and experiences so that they are better recognizable, calculable, and useful for proponents of the research program. That is, *the violent brain necessitates a specific meaning and configuration of embodiment that can inadvertently negate the richness and complexity of social living.*[3] This is both the greatest strength and the greatest weakness of the violent brain model.

Through both use and anticipation, this model *reads, forgets, and envisions* the social, or a "socialness" to warrant its role as a legitimate rubric. When employing the violent brain, researchers *read* into purpose very specific bonds between the body and social experiences, limiting both what "social experience" is supposed to look like and how it is supposed to act on and through the body. This practice projecting specific, empirically serviceable, biosocial meanings onto the model also begets the power to *forget*, or selectively abstain from, social dynamics seen as too complex or too politically volatile to claim neurobiologically knowable or valuable in neurobiological research, the most expressly visible example is demonstrated by the complexities of racism.

Finally, neuroscientists *envision* a particular promise for neurobiology through this framework: continually envisioning, or better yet conceptually mapping, a seemingly universal platform to better know and predict "susceptible subjects." This is not to imply that there is only one way to know and make "susceptible subjects," but the making and purpose of the violent brain are interlocked with a specific kind of imaginary of its intended social worth. Social assumptions and cultural slippages are built into the violent brain through these practices of reading, forgetting, and envisioning, and materialize as expected values for and vital representations of the susceptible individual.

What is made discoverable through the violent brain, then, is not necessarily a new reality about violence. As philosopher Jan De Vos states it, "What is put under the scanner is not a body, it is even not the psychological features one wants to find the neural underpinnings for; what is put under the scanner is psychological theory."[4] De Vos's critique reiterates Dumit's cogent statement that neuroscientists have maintained that the "right questions" were asked about violence in the past, but with the "wrong technologies."[5] As noted throughout this book, even at optimal use the violent brain model can fail to explicate unequivocal findings about violence. It is now clear that such slippages, inconsistences, and overall uncertainties produced through this framework may represent artifacts of past and incomplete theories of biology and violence. Moreover, it makes clear that the violent brain thesis was never just about generating biological, or biosocial, factors of violence, but always and simultaneously a sociopolitical practice: salvaging the operation of past psychological theory, defending the right to pursue biological knowledges of violence, and pushing back against critics who question its scientific validity and social purpose; intuitively, stipulating what "ought to be" *the* way to know and address violence *and* realize a normal and safe society.

THE NORMATIVITY OF THE VIOLENT BRAIN

Nikolas Rose issues a request that "we . . . pause, and . . . ask ourselves what are the benefits, and what are the dangers, of this emerging logic for the conduct of conduct: not so much 'discipline and punish,' but 'screen and intervene.'"[6] This, I believe, is directly related to unpacking the "regimes of normativity" that underpin neuroscientific research on behavior, which is never outside our understanding of violence and crime as well as safety and health.[7] Promises of the violent brain framework are inseparable from the normative expectations of the criminal. "Normative" here implies that the purpose of the violent brain is based, somewhat uncritically, on universal philosophies of "justice," "safety," and "freedom," just as much as biomedical ideals of "health" and "risk;" are unequally enforced and applied ideals that are intricately tied to regimes of power.

Neuroscientists anticipate that neurobiological knowledges will help individuals realize their agency over their own behaviors and chances for rehabilitation. Seemingly, individuals who are neurobiologically risky will be inspired to better cope with and seek treatment for their potential future violent behaviors once they are able to "see" that the cause of their aberrant actions and decisions has been their brain all along. The encouraging part about the therapeutic imaginary is that it promotes rehabilitation and prevention, presumably pushing back against blanket punitive responses to violence. Yet, the normative valence undergirding this logic undermines the transformative potentiality envisioned by neuroscientists.

Students of biopolitics will immediately recognize the parallels between this imaginary and Foucauldian "self-disciplining."[8] This model helps to cultivate and normalize a discursive sense of responsibility: individuals may gain better control of their bodies or behaviors by striving for a healthier brain. Healthy social behaviors, in this sense, are those allowable under social laws and, increasingly, those that can be authenticated neurobiologically as traits of a "healthy" or "normal" brain. Moreover, this imaginary of the violent brain fits within a framework of "technologies of security."[9] More than providing a future vision of rehabilitation, it takes its shape and operates by "finding support in the reality of the phenomenon."[10] As Lemke notes, "Rather than adjusting reality to a predefined 'should-be' value, technologies of security take reality as the norm. . . . They do not draw an absolute borderline between the permitted and the prohibited; rather they specify an optimal middle within a spectrum of variations."[11] What reality, and whose reality, do neuroscientists adopt to produce this "optimal middle"? What does it actually take to manage one's violent tendencies? The violent brain's imaginary, while carving out a version of what "ought to be," is also made through and preserves, or will help normalize, the purpose and function of certain social ideals and truisms.

The risk of neurobiological understandings of violence lies in its plausibility in the larger society. Society is not, and will not be, a passive observer in this contemporary rendering of biology and violence. In fact, specific publics may be more curious, convinced by, and invested in the prospect of uncovering a biological influence of violence than neuroscientists are. As these understandings of the violent brain are incorporated, albeit unevenly, within society they will likely latch on to, and not undermine or replace, existing discourses of power. Normalization anticipates flexibility, according to Canguilhem: "So, we see how a technological norm gradually reflects an idea of society and its hierarchy of values, how a decision to normalize assumes the representation of a possible whole of correlative, complementary or compensatory decision. This whole must be finished in advance, finished if not closed."[12] This reflexive characteristic makes such models serviceable for a variety of different social worlds, flexible and "normal" enough to help the psychiatrist ascertain a patient's psychopathic risk or to help the judge understand the violent offender's actions before rendering judgment.

While it is unclear whether the larger public buys, or will buy, the claim that crime is the result of a "broken brain," it is realistic to consider that the violent brain, and this model's aim of picturing distinctive and innate risks for deviancy at an individual level, will produce and rationalize rhetoric concerning self-control, personal responsibility, and social insecurity that then helps justify mechanisms of social control for violence or criminality. Like biomedical understandings of violence, existing criminal justice or penal institutions have also been less devoted to delineating, or enacting, the precise qualities of the criminal or crime in any outright manner. The investment in and rise of the U.S. carceral state are best explained as functions of the mounting "social insecurities" in the latter half of the twentieth century rather than as a reaction to amassing criminal behavior, argues sociologist Loïc Wacquant.[13] These policies and practices concurrently enclose violent and criminal behaviors in a frame of personal choice or wrong decisions, an inability to manage one's violent or antisocial tendencies. A neurobiological understanding of violence also functions through a logic of individual choice, albeit with a biomedical justification. Thus the violent brain model tries to create an avenue for individual change, a promise that rests on the encouragement of brain-based management of violence, if only one can first recognize, and adhere to, the neurobiological risk.

It is unsurprising, then, that defense lawyers have been open to using neurobiological knowledges as proof of their clients' predisposition to violence, as the larger legal system has encouraged them to exhaust all avenues to keep a client off of death row.[14] Despite the very real possibility that the violent brain may also indicate that such individuals are "incurable," having brains that may help predict their future transgression but that will require continual intervention and management of neurobiological risk. Legal scholar Michelle Alexander reminds us that "the nature of the criminal justice system has changed. It is no longer concerned primarily with the prevention and punishment of crime, but rather with the management and control of the dispossessed."[15] Alexander's words seem to suggest that the criminal justice system is eerily primed for a seamless adoption of "screen and intervene," as it necessitates the management and control of risk, similar to requirements for the susceptible individual under the violent brain model.

Neurobiological knowledges of violence, in this sense, represent technoscientific corroboration of a particularly "reality." While biomarkers for violent traits may be rationalized as signs of mental distress in some social groups, they will simultaneously help to harden stereotypes of and discrimination against "others," providing unequivocal neurobiological proof that some cultural or racial groups naturally possess and express tendencies for violent, antisocial, or abnormal behaviors or tastes. At the same time, the violent brain also works for those individuals or institutions that genuinely desire better, maybe more creative, solutions to violence, as the current (social) policies just are not working or are too politically biased or economically strapped to make effective changes. These segments of society are hopeful, if not assured, that the technological savviness of the neurosciences will yield greater facts about and substantial solutions to violence. Thus, biological ideas of violence will remain viable not just because of advances in biotechnologies of behavior, but also because of society's own pervasive and rather dogmatic inclination to view criminals as natural "kinds" of humans, seemingly distinct from normal individuals as a result of supposed intrinsic deficiencies or motivations that make them independently accountable for their own (mis)behavior.

"RE-READING" THE VIOLENT BRAIN

What does it imply that a violent brain framework "works" optimally, in a more realizable and likely more comprehensible fashion, *absent* the consideration of sociocultural complexity, inequality, and power? What if the laboratory setbacks of this model are showing neuroscientists something different? Warning them of the limits to this biosocial configuration, and the desires to explain our behaviors in terms of cortical thickness, neurochemical pathways, or actual neuronal firing patterns? The violent brain's inconsistences, those moments when neuroscientific "intuition" tells neuroscientists that this technology has reached its limits, could be the flashing sirens imploring them to pay closer attention to the things that this model cannot do—what the neuroscience of behavior has not done. Thus, we need to interrogate the "weakness," "fragility," and limits of the neurosciences, instead of assuming that such practices operate from a position of strength.[16]

Neuroscientists anticipate a greater chance for a more just, safe, and free society. It is, though, more likely that true social function of the violent brain model will support existing criminal polices that are more punitive than rehabilitative, and that will actively restructure and deprive provisions of social support and security.[17] This alternative appraisal of the violent brain construct views its failures as the signs of a normative valence. Careful attention to how emotional, strategic, and corrective meanings appear within this technical framework makes it clear that sociocultural dynamics and discourses should challenge its abilities to "work" as designed. This assessment draws attention to its *lack* of social imagination and ingenuity. This is not an indication of empirical ineptness, but a clue that certain social meanings, complexities, and lives are being meticulously overlooked and erased from these biosocial equations of life. It is not enough to accept that neurobiological knowledges have an inherent ethical function, which supposedly will prevent them from legitimating social deficits and inequalities that already exist.

A biopolitics of the violent brain is unavoidable given that its object of study, violence, intuitively straddles the political, moral, and legal social worlds. The power of biopolitics "lies in its ability to make visible the always contingent, always precarious difference between politics and life, culture and nature, between the realm of the intangible and unquestioned, on the one hand, and the sphere of moral and legal action, on the other."[18] The intent of the neuroscientists may not be the central problem inasmuch as the violent brain construct, like other sociocultural technologies and prac- tices today, is built through existing ideologies that help to "ensure a space for extending socio-racial interventions" with or without purpose.[19] To this point, inequality must be at the heart of a biopolitics of the violent brain; thus for social scientists this is not just a rereading of the violent brain model but a refocusing of biopolitics in order to illuminate scientific inabilities to address inequity.[20]

Reassesing the place of inequality in this model of violence may lead neuroscientists to rethink the ambition of "predicting" violence, as that may not be the most optimal way to prevent such actions or keep society safe. A rereading of the violent brain takes seriously the fact that predicting violence can never be devoid of political and moral morass, which neuroscientists opt to surpass, or suppress, through a neurobiological framework of risk. This is tacitly acknowledged by some neuroscientists already, who insist that the violent brain model be limited to clinical populations, yet its promise remains bound to its anticipated utility upon normal and healthy population just as much as clinical ones. A rereading may also show that the histories and sociality read through our brains (or genes) require us to take more seriously the way we organize and conceptualize the categories within society that we call "criminal," "sick," and "abnormal," leading us toward greater focus on the socioculturally embedded cumulative disadvantages that may elude the molecular level. Since neurobiological interpretations of crime seek to delineate unique brain signatures in at-risk populations early enough (if not asymptomatically) in order to decrease the chance that members of those groups develop mental disorders, such interpretations are increasingly expanding the bounds of who can be at risk, and what should count as a potential risk factor. There is a universalism to the violent brain: the construct produces a unique type of "patient," but also posits that anyone can be neurobiologically vulnerable for violence. Thus, scientific "[p]erspectives are not ways to 'approach' a nature that is already there; instead, the intersection of perspectives stratifies nature and makes it meaningful."[21] The point here is to illuminate what empirical flexibility allows researchers to forget or reimagine when employing this framework, not to deny entanglements between bodies and social experiences.

One of the most striking things about the violent brain model is how my own life experiences, particularly the navigation of race/racism in society, lie outside of its inquiry. Though the violent brain construct is presented as a more plastic, race-neutral, and technologically advanced explanation for violence, there is little proof that social power can be unpacked and interrogated through the etiological logic applied in this model. For an African American male, like myself, this lack of proof may at first seem to be a relief, a chance to avoid the limits and potential mistakes of this technology, which turns out not to be flexible enough to read all minds. The idea that race is no longer a direct focus of the biology of violence, however, provides no real assurance that neurobiological knowledges of violence will help alleviate or lessen the ways in which the citizenship rights and societal worth of racially marginalized populations are constantly being devalued, undermined, or outright ignored in order to maintain ideals of safety and freedom. Thus, racism may be too complex for this technology to handle, but its omission does not prevent the violent brain from functioning as a "color-blind technology."[22] The existing enactment of the violent brain implicitly denies the reality of complex racial dynamics and the racializing work of biological discourses that are always already embedded in the social practices of violence—the way we recognize, "know," and anticipate who is violent.

If the violent brain is incapable of providing a meaningful biosocial understanding of the way racism shapes, and is shaped by, violence in society, then how is it supposed to envision a realistic understanding of my neurobiological risk? How can it reckon with the lives of the socially marginalized, whose experiences are placed outside, or counter to, normative notions of citizenship and responsibility, who hold a rational reluctance to trust the wheels of justice or scientific progress? Even if I knew my own neurobiological risks for violence (and for the record, I do not know them, nor would I want to know), that knowledge would seem incomplete, detached from my reality, in which the social practice of race reveals to U.S. society how to think about my potential dangerousness even before I'm able to introduce myself.

Rereading the violent brain is not to reject a role of the prefrontal cortex in behavior or to doubt that the amygdala really did "light up" during an experiment. It is rather to understand the type of violent brain interpretation that is likely for those questions, experiences, and social bodies that escape neuroscientific intuition. For example, if violence is a result of the brain's inabilities, how does the violent brain make sense of the social spaces in which such failures provide a positive function? The brain's inabilities to hinder violent tendencies present as social assets in socially sanctioned arenas of violent entertainment (i.e., boxing, mixed-martial arts, or American football), or through state-authorized institutions in society (i.e., police or military). These social spaces are not conceptualized by the violent brain as the "negative environments" facilitating unwanted neurochemical activity. In the case of policing, more specifically, it seems unlikely that the current configuration of the violent brain will provide a realistic explanation for the rampant police shootings of African Americans or the persistent surveillance and suspicion of Arab and Muslim populations. Moreover, institutional policies defend, protect, and license the police to "stop and frisk," physically restrain, or shoot individuals considered risky due to nothing more than their race or ethnicity; these are social pressures that law enforcement is asked to face and the societal authority it is expected to embody. However, such practices, or politics, of race are the types of "social" that do not fit under the scanner. A rereading of the violent brain model, then, requires reevaluating what a biosocial variable really means or does for our understanding of violence in a purposely intended racially unequal social landscape. This also necessitates a refocusing of biopolitics to anticipate when and how a neurobiological construct like the violent brain, through its optimal capabilities and auto-mated functionality, *reads, forgets, and envisions* meaning and purpose in bodies and brains like mine.

Social inequality, while not the focus of the violent brain, is not challenged through its function, and may become more entrenched as a means of taking the biological-social nexus seriously without challenging the sociopolitical systemic practices and institutions that help engender "unequal lives" in society. "The most basic recognition owed to those who bear the weight of the inequality of lives is to recognize not only this reality but also the consistent denial of it, a denial of which they themselves are acutely aware."[23] An un-derstanding of the social implications, the social anticipation, of the violent brain must abandon taking the "objective" or normalized view as a starting point; instead it must embrace a purposeful subjective *standpoint* that takes seriously the inseparable relationship between a society's views and experi-ences of violence and its dependency on stratified life chances.[24] Without this reframing, a biopolitics of the violent brain may work no differently than the construct itself, increasing the chance that it will, willing or not, reproduce the ethical dilemmas that it was supposedly built to address, and engender newer, even more complicated repercussions for social issues that critics are hoping to avoid. Thus, as neuroscientists eagerly strive to unlock the secrets to violence that are seemingly hidden away in our brains, we must ask: At what cost? And more crucially, At *whose* cost?

Notes

PREFACE

1. Williams, Lawrence, and Davis, "Racism and Health"; Phelan and Link, "Is Racism a Fundamental Cause of Inequalities in Health?"

2. Heron, "Deaths: Leading Causes for 2017."

3. Fullwiley, "The Molecularization of Race."

4. Roberts, *Fatal Invention*.

5. Koenig, Lee, and Richardson, *Revisiting Race in a Genomic Age*; Fujimura, Duster, and Rajagopalan, "Introduction: Race, Genetics, and Disease"; Wailoo, Nelson, and Lee, *Genetics and the Unsettled Past*; Whitmarsh and Jones, *What's the Use of Race?*; Bliss, *Race Decoded*.

6. Uttal, *The New Phrenology*; Friston, "Beyond Phrenology"; Kosik, "Beyond Phrenology, at Last"; Donaldson, "Parsing Brain Activity"; Diener, "Neuroimaging"; Cornel, "Something Old, Something New, Something Pseudo, Something True."

7. Duster, "Comparative Perspectives and Competing Explanations."

8. Alexander, *The New Jim Crow*; Anderson, *Code of the Street*; Gabbidon, *Criminological Perspectives on Race and Crime*; Muhammad, *The Condemnation of Blackness*; Pinderhughes, *Race in the Hood*; Rios, *Punished*; Ward, "The Slow Violence of State Organized Race Crime."

9. This is a relatively small group of scientists, and the names of all participants were changed to protect the identity of the neuroscientists and their labs. The study was approved through UCSF's internal review board.

10. The term "color-blind racism" is used to critique the ideology/practice that ignoring race or avoiding "race-talk" is the best way to combat racism. To ignore race is not to be "racist" per se, but it can signal a failure to account for the intricate ways in which racial meaning and consequences more often operate covertly, without need for direct gesture, acknowledgment, or specificity. In *Racism without Racists*, Eduardo Bonilla-Silva argues that color-blind racism hides the true nature of race/racism in society. Racism is treated as a rare and individualized behavior or mentality, instead of as an array of systemic practices that have been embedded—historically, culturally, and politically—in everyday social dynamics and institutions. See also Brown et al., *Whitewashing Race*; Obasogie, *Blinded by Sight*; Ray and Purifoy, "The Colorblind Organization"; Burke, *Colorblind Racism*.

11. Kuhn, *The Structure of Scientific Revolutions*; Fleck, *Genesis and Development of a Scientific Fact*; Latour and Woolgar, *Laboratory Life*; Shapin and Schaffer, *Leviathan and the Air-Pump*.

12. Du Bois, *The Souls of Black Folk*, 13.

13. Du Bois, *The Souls of Black Folk*.

14. Jasanoff, "The Idiom of Co-Production."

15. Benjamin, "Innovating Inequity."

16. Duster, *Backdoor to Eugenics*; Duster, "Explaining Differential Trust"; Duster, "Lessons from History"; Duster, "Behavioral Genetics and the Link between Crime, Violence, and Race."

CHAPTER 1

1. Herbert, "Politics of Biology," 72. Earlier works on the social, cultural, and ethical impacts of the gene in the 1990s, specifically Duster's *Backdoor to Eugenics* and Nelkin and Lindee's *The DNA Mystique*, provide meticulous examinations of the brief arguments presented in Herbert's commentary.

2. Herbert, "Politics of Biology."

3. Herbert, "Politics of Biology," 79.

4. Rafter, *The Criminal Brain*.

5. Duster, *Backdoor to Eugenics*; Wasserman and Wachbroit, *Genetics and Criminal Behavior*; Marsh and Katz, *Biology, Crime and Ethics*.

6. Rose, *The Politics of Life Itself*.

7. Panofsky, *Misbehaving Science*, 177.

8. Allen, "Old Wine in New Bottles."

9. Nelkin and Lindee, *The DNA Mystique*.

10. Nelkin and Lindee, 2.

11. Duster, "Lessons from History"; Rensberger, "Science and Sensitivity"; Anderson, "NIH, under Fire, Freezes Grant for Conference on Genetics and Crime."

12. There is a problematic history of tying race to intelligence, and such knowledges have been utilized in research on the biology of violence to emphasize links among race, intelligence, and criminal behavior. See Gould, *The Mismeasure of Man*. Moreover, concerns about race and the genetics of crime continued in the following decade, with the completion of the Human Genome Project (HGP) and the expanding dependency on DNA forensic technologies. See also Duster, "Explaining Differential Trust"; Larregue and Rollins, "Biosocial Criminology and the Mismeasure of Race"; M'charek, "Silent Witness, Articulate Collective"; Ossorio and Duster, "Race and Genetics"; Prainsack and Kitzberger, "DNA behind Bars"; Rollins, "Risky Bodies."

13. Duster, "Explaining Differential Trust"; Prainsack and Kitzberger, "DNA behind Bars"; M'charek, "Silent Witness, Articulate Collective"; Greely et al., "Family Ties"; Rollins, "Risky Bodies."

14. Bush, "Decade of the Brain: Presidential Proclamation 6158"; Obama, "Remarks by the President on the BRAIN Initiative and American Innovation."

15. Dana Foundation, "A Decade after the Decade of the Brain: Compilation"; Volkow, Koob, and McLellan, "Neurobiologic Advances from the Brain Disease Model of Addiction."

16. Lieberman, *Social*.

17. "Brainhood, Anthropological Figure of Modernity." "Brainhood" is defined by Fernando Vidal (2009, 6) as "the property or quality of being, rather than simply having, a brain."

18. Neuroscience departments are rather recent; thus the "neuroscience community" represents a diverse number of disciplines all converging on a "neuro-molecular style of thought." Rose and Abi-Rached, *Neuro*.

19. For examples, see Abigail Marsh's work on altruism, *The Fear Factor*. For childhood development and maltreatment, see the work of Essi Viding and Eamon McCory et al., e.g., "Neurocognitive Adaptation and Mental Health Vulnerability following Maltreatment"; and the work from Luke Hyde's lab, Gard et al., "The Long Reach of Early Adversity."

20. Lakatos, "Falsification and the Methodology of Scientific Research Programmes"; see also Hacking, "Degeneracy, Criminal Behavior, and Looping," 144–45.

21. Hacking derived this characterization from philosopher of science Imre Lakatos's *research programme*. See Lakatos, "Falsification and the Methodology of Scientific Research Programmes." In the Lakatosian sense, a *research programme* "can last a century or more, and [is] characterized not by investigators with proposals, but by a sequence of theories (Ts) . . . [which] share a *hard core* of basic and unquestioned hypothesis; successive Ts result from previous Ts by modifying the *protective belt* of auxiliary hypotheses." "Degeneracy, Criminal Behavior,

and Looping," 144. Like Hacking, I agree that Lakatos's argument is less useful for most modes of science, but that it does serve to help us better understand the sustained endurance, and proclaimed usefulness, of the biology of violence.

22. Hacking, "Degeneracy, Criminal Behavior, and Looping," 145.

23. Degenerate theories of crime have been a key principle in much of criminology research. However, not all theories have focused on individual degeneracy, and for others degeneracy has not been a useful starting point at all. Some sociological theories of crime have shifted attention away from individuals (criminals or violent offenders) and toward social institutions, spaces, and conditions. Moreover, others have been less focused on degeneracy as a throwback to former human kind, or a lack in moral fabric of a civilization that once was. Instead, more-critical criminological perspectives—feminist, antiracist, anticolonial, and/or Marxist—reject recovering a normative "what was" or contemplating the "atypical," in order to promote a more-critical understanding of the limits of existing criminal theories and structures in society, and the way they have capitalized on power and inequality.

24. In Lakatos's formulation, the protective belt is thought to arise from additional, or *auxiliary, hypotheses*, core beliefs that function heuristically. The protective belt continually revises, reshapes, and reformulates the core beliefs of a science to help refute antagonistic facts or theories, thus insulating the program and helping to preserve its hard core. Lakatos, "Falsification and the Methodology of Scientific Research Programmes."

25. Rose, *The Politics of Life Itself*, 242.

26. Rose, 242.

27. Niehoff, *The Biology of Violence*, 5.

28. Vidal, "What Makes Neuroethics Possible?," 1.

29. Vidal, 1 (emphasis added).

30. Coproduction here draws from Sheila Jasanoff's "The Idiom of Co-Production," 2. Jasanoff explains that coproduction captures that "the ways in which we know and represent the world (both nature and society) are inseparable from the ways in which we choose to live in it."

31. Beckwith, "The Persistent Influence of Failed Scientific Ideas."

32. Panofsky, *Misbehaving Science*, 9.

33. Rose and Abi-Rached, *Neuro*, 29.

34. The use of "work" here draws from Star and Strauss's arguments about "articulation work" or "invisible work," although I would not go so far as to say that the program's history is articulation work. Instead, the labor here refers to a specific reflexivity between the researcher and research practices. Susan L. Star and Anselm Strauss argue that articulation work "gets things back 'on track' in

the face of the unexpected, and modifies action to accommodate unanticipated contingencies. The important thing about articulation work is that it is invisible to rationalized models of work." Star and Strauss, "Layers of Silence, Arenas of Voice," 10.

35. The names of the neuroscientists I interviewed have all been changed to pseudonyms.

36. Hacking, "Degeneracy, Criminal Behavior, and Looping."

37. Pickersgill, "Ordering Disorder"; Star, *Regions of the Mind*.

38. Niehoff, *The Biology of Violence*, 30.

39. Adolphs, "The Social Brain"; Blakemore, "The Social Brain in Adolescence"; Frith, "The Social Brain?"; Lieberman, *Social*.

40. Niehoff, *The Biology of Violence*, 260.

41. Dupras and Ravitsky, "Epigenetics in the Neoliberal 'Regime of Truth,'" 31.

42. Rose, *The Politics of Life Itself*, 70.

43. Castel, "From Dangerousness to Risk."

44. Castel, 281.

45. Rose, "'Screen and Intervene.'"

46. The work of anthropologist Joseph Dumit is particularly important here. Dumit has demonstrated how neuroimaging acts as a techno-social rubric to help facilitate "objective self-fashioning" For him, the remaking of personhood through this process increases the cultural authority of the neurosciences. See *Picturing Personhood*. Similarly, Vidal also theorizes about the "cerebral subject" as an anthropological figure characterized by "the property or quality of *being*, rather than simply *having*, a brain." He sees this ideology as the ontological catalyst for neuroscientific investigations into social and cultural worlds. Vidal's work asks, or rather requests, that we probe what kinds of narratives of "the self" the "cerebral subject" necessitates to justify its making, existence, and potential in society. See "Brainhood, Anthropological Figure of Modernity."

47. Dumit, *Picturing Personhood*.

48. Fassin, *Life*.

49. Harcourt, "Risk as a Proxy for Race," 237.

50. Dumit, *Picturing Personhood*; Rose, *The Politics of Life Itself*.

51. James, Resisting State Violence, 26–28.

52. Adams, Murphy, and Clarke, "Anticipation."

53. Mills, *The Sociological Imagination*.

54. M'charek, Schramm, and Skinner, "Technologies of Belonging." "Absent presence" is "something that oscillates between reality and nonreality, which appears on the surface and then hides underground." "Absent presence" helps situate the way race informs different scientific practices and how race-based

identities are made and reconstituted through biomedical technologies. See also Karkazis and Jordan-Young's "Sensing Race as a Ghost Variable in Science, Technology, and Medicine."

55. Muhammad, *The Condemnation of Blackness*. Muhammad introduces this phrase in chapter 2 (35–87) to show how racial statistics, in the sciences and social sciences, have been historically (mis)used to create a seemingly rational depiction of "black crime." However, Muhammad's entire book can be read as a successful interrogation of concept, including its salience in the present day.

56. Rubin, "Therapeutic Promise."

57. Pickersgill, "Between Soma and Society."

58. My argument here draws from Didier Fassin's *Life* and Alexander Weheliye's *Habeas Viscus*. Both provide convincing arguments that challenge us to re-analyze, if not fully discard, classic notions of biopolitics. Instead, their work centers on inequality (Fassin) and "racializing assembleges" (Weheliye) in order to provide a more lucid and productive understanding of the politics of human life.

CHAPTER 2

1. The biology of violence can be divided into roughly three stages: the "born criminal" era led by the work of Lombroso to turn criminology into a recognizable academic discipline (late 1800s to 1945); the medicalization era (1960s to 1980s); and the biomedicalization era (late 1990s to the present). Here, I draw from the analysis of Adele Clarke and her colleagues describing the transformations of medicine in the twentieth century; see Clarke, Mamo et al., *Biomedicalization*, chapter 2. Although the biology of violence has not always been framed in strict medical or biomedical terms, the return of biocriminology from the mid-1960s to the emergence of the molecular era (~ late 1980s) mirrors the transformations captured in Clarke, Mamo et al.'s meticulous examination of modern medicine.

2. These eras in the biology of violence are not mutually exclusive; as noted above. The origins of thinking about mental abilities and criminality that predominated during the medicalization era stretched back to at least the 1930s. Heredity research on violence can also be dated to this period in Germany, and the use of twin and family studies remains a staple in behavioral genetics of violence in the biomedicalization era. The application of these eras helps explain how and why today's researchers anchor their beliefs in this research program, that they are capable of achieving something different than in the past, but it also provides a way to relationally map the specific ontological commitments that continue to shape the program today. That is, these eras situate the book to

approach and analyze the properties of conviction that go into the defense of today's biology of violence in its neuroscientific form.

3. Rafter, "H. J. Eysenck in Fagin's Kitchen," 38. To be clear, biological theories of violence never disappeared completely. While sociological theories garnered the majority of support, biological influences on behavior remained as well; see also Rafter, *The Criminal Brain*.

4. Eysenck stated that personality was the product of two intersecting dimensions: emotional state dimension (ranging from stable to unstable or liability) and a scale of extraversion-introversion. In subsequent editions, he eventually changed this statement to (1) reflect an understanding of criminals who could be introverts and have low-level emotions and (2) add a third dimension to his theory, psychoticism.

5. Here, Eysenck relied on genetic research focused on twins, intelligence, and criminal behavior to make the argument that conditioning was tied to heredity. He also argued that criminals tended to have lower intelligence, and that intelligence, like personality, was hereditary. He briefly alluded to neuroscience, specifically neurophysiology, research that focused on brain structure. He used this literature to argue that the reticular formation (RF) area of the brain acted as a gatekeeper, allowing information to pass between the brain and the rest of the body. Eysenck was trying to point out that RF was part of the automatic nervous system, and that this physiological system was active in the conditioning process and therefore responsible for controlling our emotions. The reticular formation (RF) is a bundle of nerves that runs along the length of the brain stem (area of the brain that connects the brain to the spinal cord). In terms of evolution, it is considered one of the oldest parts of the anatomy, and therefore is said to control the most basic functions of the body (i.e., the automatic nervous system, such as heartbeat or sleep cycles).

6. The medicalization era of the biology of violence included heredity research on the possible genetic contributions of violence (e.g., twin and XYY chromosomal studies), neurophysiological research on antisocial criminality and psychopathy; and controversial psychosurgery treatments to "cure" uncontrollable violent or aggressive tendencies in mentally ill criminal populations.

7. Boffey, Carter, and Hamilton, "Nixon Budget"; Coleman, "Perspectives on the Medical Research of Violence."

8. Coleman, "Perspectives on the Medical Research of Violence," 675.

9. Coleman, "Perspectives on the Medical Research of Violence"; Conrad and Schneider, *Deviance and Medicalization*; Moran, "Biomedical Research and the Politics of Crime Control."

10. Conrad and Schneider, *Deviance and Medicalization*.

11. Chorover, "Violence," 260.

12. Clarke, Shim et al., "Biomedicalization."

13. Clarke, Mamo et al., *Biomedicalization*.

14. Clarke, Mamo et al., 57–82, outlined five key overlapping processes that can be used to better elucidate biomedicalization: (1) new biopolitical economy of medicine; (2) intensified focus on health and risk, and surveillance; (3) technoscientization of biomedical practices; (4) transformation of biomedical knowledge production; and (5) transformation of bodies and the production of new identities.

15. Duster, "Behavioral Genetics and the Link between Crime, Violence, and Race," 153.

16. Duster, 156.

17. Bufkin and Luttrell, "Neuroimaging Studies of Aggressive and Violent Behavior," 177.

18. The Aspen Neurobehavioral Conference (ANC) convened for two sessions in the late 1990s. The ANC was an annual conference on issues related to mind and brain, and the consensus statement was the result of the meetings' findings on neurobiology and violence. The group's participants represented neurology, neuropsychology, psychiatry, trauma surgery, nursing, evolutionary psychology, medical ethics, and law.

19. Volavka, *Neurobiology of Violence*.

20. Loeber and Pardini, "Neurobiology and the Development of Violence," 1 (emphasis added).

21. Kiehl, *The Psychopath Whisperer*.

22. Randy J. Nelson, *Biology of Aggression*, v.

23. Star, *Regions of the Mind*, 16.

24. In this book, "*DSM*" refers to *DSM-IV*. Although *DSM-V* (2013) is the current version, the bulk of articles reviewed in this volume were published before *DSM-V* was released.

25. This class of personality disorders is also outlined in *The International Classification of Diseases* (*ICD*), the psychological classification manual sponsored by the World Health Organization (WHO). The studies I reviewed cited the *ICD* less frequently than the *DSM*, but the criteria for several of the personality disorders associated with violence are quite similar; although the names are not always the same, the *ICD* uses the term "dissocial personality disorder" instead of "antisocial personality disorder."

26. Fishbein, *Biobehavioral Perspectives on Criminology*.

27. Hacking, "Degeneracy, Criminal Behavior, and Looping"; Pickersgill, "Standardising Antisocial Personality Disorder."

28. Biosocial criminology has emerged as a sub-discipline of criminology. These researchers have utilized findings from the neurobiology of violence in an effort to improve the accuracy and efficacy of criminological theory. See Beaver, *Biosocial Criminology*. However, many of the new claims about the genetic or neuroscientific basis of crime rely on antiquated evolutionary notions of race and refuted understandings of the heritability of crime. For a review of social and ethical critiques of this subfield, see Larregue, *Héréditaire*; Carrier and Walby, "Ptolemizing Lombroso"; Larregue and Rollins, "Biosocial Criminology and the Mismeasure of Race"; Burt and Simons, "Pulling Back the Curtain on Heritability Studies."

29. Interview, Dr. Lewis, 10/7/11.

30. Pickersgill, "The Endurance of Uncertainty," 143.

31. Star, *Regions of the Mind*.

32. Raine, *The Psychopathology of Crime*, 3 (emphasis added).

33. Bowker and Star, *Sorting Things Out*; Timmermans and Epstein, "A World of Standards but Not a Standard World."

34. Pickersgill, "The Endurance of Uncertainty," 143.

35. Blake and Grafman, "The Neurobiology of Aggression," 12.

36. Epstein, "The Rise of 'Recruitmentology,'" 801 (emphasis added).

37. Following Bourdieu's analysis of cultural and symbolic capital, Panofsky notes that "scientific capital is the meeting point of the field of forces and struggles—it is the object of competition whose accumulation and distribution are crucial forces." Panofsky, "Field Analysis and Interdisciplinary Science," 295–96. Scientific capital, then, is an extension of symbolic capital, a form of social power that is based on the scientific authority, technical legitimation, and a perceived command over and accumulation of knowledge. See also Bourdieu, "The Specificity of the Scientific Field and the Social Conditions of the Progress of Reason."

38. Kiehl, *The Psychopath Whisperer*, 124 (emphasis in original).

39. Kiehl contributed to each phase of building the MRI machine, but this prep work included the coordination of correction offices, and the corporation and labor of prisoners. His unit would differ from the one that nearly ran him off the road. It required unique computer engineering, technological specifications, and electrical power because it would be used to capture functional images of the brain. This project also needed more-complex safety measures, since it would be transportable and used on a population of violent offenders that already required special precautions. Moreover, changes to the prison's operations and structure were also required to host a state-of-the-art multimillion-dollar magnet. Kiehl recalls the facility director of one prison talking to him about the site where the machine would be parked: "I had the inmates build the concrete pad and dig

the road along the back of the medical wing. The electrician was able to trench out the connections. So we are all set" (Kiehl, 182). Kiehl's staff would work out of the medical wing once in a prison, and the machine would be parked there for a set amount of time, in order to maximize the lab's research potential to recruit and scan a greater number of inmates who exhibited psychopathic traits.

40. Neurotechnologies have also produced new strategies of recruitmentology, and as shown below, these strategies have allowed researchers to move beyond incarcerated populations. Nevertheless, Kiehl's mobile MRI is often regarded as a benchmark for best assisting in recruitment of important populations. Kiehl was always going to need access to this important population to do his work. However, his efforts were supported in part by the enthusiasm among university, state, and prison officials about scanning the brains of inmates and the potential of finding out more about why they are violent, and the use of this technology helped to convince both prison officials and prisoners that participating in this study was worthwhile.

41. Fishbein, *Biobehavioral Perspectives on Criminology*, 12 (emphasis added).

42. American Psychiatric Association, *Diagnostic and Statistical Manual of Mental Disorders*.

43. Two personality disorders that have been linked to violence through neuroimaging and genetic studies were excluded from my analysis—schizophrenia and borderline personality disorder—because neither requires the presence of violent or aggressive behavior for diagnosis.

44. Frick and Viding, "Antisocial Behavior from a Developmental Psychopathology Perspective"; Viding and McCrory, "Why Should We Care about Measuring Callous-Unemotional Traits in Children?"

45. Holmes and Patrick, "The Myth of Optimality in Clinical Neuroscience," 241.

46. Fishbein, *Biobehavioral Perspectives on Criminology*, 12 (emphasis added).

47. American Psychiatric Association, *Diagnostic and Statistical Manual of Mental Disorders*, 4th ed., text rev., 93.

48. Coccaro, "Intermittent Explosive Disorder."

49. American Psychiatric Association, *Diagnostic and Statistical Manual of Mental Disorders*, 4th ed., text rev.,706.

50. Pickersgill, "The Endurance of Uncertainty"; Pickersgill, "Standardising Antisocial Personality Disorder."

51. Interview, Dr. Smith, 5/7/12.

52. Blair, "Psychopathy."

53. Health (UK), *Antisocial Personality Disorder*; Hare, "The Hare PCL-R";

Ogloff, "Psychopathy/Antisocial Personality Disorder Conundrum"; Lynam and Vachon, "Antisocial Personality Disorder in DSM-5."

54. Pickersgill, "NICE Guidelines, Clinical Practice and Antisocial Personality Disorder."

55. Pickersgill, "Standardising Antisocial Personality Disorder," 545.

56. Pickersgill, "Standardising Antisocial Personality Disorder."

57. Malterer et al., "Concurrent Validity of the Psychopathic Personality Inventory with Offender and Community Samples."

58. Ly et al., "Cortical Thinning in Psychopathy."

59. Anderson and Kiehl, "The Psychopath Magnetized."

60. Blais, Forth, and Hare, "Examining the Interrater Reliability of the Hare Psychopathy Checklist." To be clear, the team noted that "interrater reliability of the PCL–R Total score and both factors were considered good, however, they fell short of a more stringent definition of "acceptable."

61. Porter, *Trust in Numbers*, 200.

62. Lemke, *Biopolitics*, 47.

63. Clarke and Casper, "From Simple Technology to Complex Arena," 614.

64. Hacking, The Social Construction of What?

65. Berkowitz, *Aggression*.

66. Blair, "Neuroimaging of Psychopathy and Antisocial Behavior."

CHAPTER 3

1. Caplan, *The Insanity Defense and the Trial of John W. Hinckley, Jr.*

2. Kevles, *Naked to the Bone*. See also Dumit, *Picturing Personhood*; Shen, "The Overlooked History of Neurolaw Symposium." Hinckley's case was one of the earliest to use CT scans in the court. Dumit, however, notes that X-rays were used as early as 1896. And legal scholar Francis Shen states that EEG (electroencephalography) evidence helped shape laws around epilepsy in the 1930s.

3. Taylor Jr., "Judge Rebukes Hinckley Witness over Cat Scan," 13.

4. Kiernan, "Hinckley Judge Reverses Himself, Admits Pictures of Defendant's Brain."

5. Dumit, *Picturing Personhood*, 112.

6. Kevles, *Naked To The Bone*; Gunderman, *X-Ray Vision*.

7. Taylor Jr., "Cat Scans Said to Show Shrunken Hinckley Brain"; Taylor, "Hinckley's Brain Is Termed Normal." In the June 4 article, prosecution witness radiologist David Davis directly rebutted testimony from the defense's expert witnesses that claimed Hinckley's brain was abnormal. Davis was quoted as saying, "Atrophy is not a disease; it's an event"; "Hinckley's Brain Is Termed Normal," 21.

8. Rose and Abi-Rached, *Neuro*.

9. Gazzaniga, "What Is Cognitive Neuroscience?," 3.

10. Joyce, *Magnetic Appeal*.

11. Aguirre, "Functional Neuroimaging." Aguirre, somewhat wary of the democratization of imaging, connects the phenomenon to the variable quality of neuroimaging research during the early 2000s.

12. Aguirre, "Functional Neuroimaging, S18.

13. Dolan, "Neuroimaging of Cognition," 497. The pervasiveness and authority of imaging research on violence, like other forms of scientific knowledge, cannot be captured by an assessment of scientific merit alone. Aguirre's and Dolan's critiques concerning the technical aptitude of "non-experts" focus too heavily on the disciplinary background, which understates the social exchanges that are imbued through research networks. This is not to dismiss Aguirre's and Dolan's warnings about the overuse and uncritical appraisals of neuroimaging, but to imply that a more salient social critique must include the kinds of work that go into imaging practices and their products beyond a researcher's qualifications. Neuroimaging research often involves a multidisciplinary network of researchers—primary investigators, graduate students, lab technicians—specializing in a range of skills beyond neuropsychology, from radiology to computer graphics. The multiplicity of expertise is vital in order for the team to properly engage and use imaging technologies and to produce and interpret the results. See Latour and Woolgar, *Laboratory Life*; Alač, "Working with Brain Scans"; Beaulieu, "Images Are Not the (Only) Truth"; Joyce, *Magnetic Appeal*.

14. Halpern, "The Neuroscience of Picking a Presidential Candidate."

15. Clarke and Fujimura, *The Right Tools for the Job*.

16. Berman, *Creating the Market University*; Gläser and Laudel, "Governing Science."

17. Philipps and Weißenborn, "Unconventional Ideas Conventionally Arranged," 893.

18. Hackett, "Funding and Academic Research in the Life Sciences," 134.

19. This does not include the 60-plus reviews and meta-analyses on the topic that have been published since 2000. The total number here is limited to neuroimaging research on personality disorders thought to be associated with violence. This total excludes studies on suicide, traumatic brain injury, schizophrenia and violent behavior, bipolar disorder and violent behavior, substance abuse, video gaming, and studies not published in English. Studies that used both functional and structural MRI techniques were counted as part of the functional imaging studies because the main findings were often framed in terms of brain function.

20. Dumit, *Picturing Personhood*, 177 (emphasis added).

21. Horn, "Making Criminologists," 320.

22. Interview, Dr. Hollowell, 10/29/11.

23. Joyce, "Neuroimaging Production in Clinical Practice," 82. "Docile patients" refers to Foucault's notion of "docile bodies."

24. Interview, Dr. Holmes, 10/4/12.

25. See Weisberg et al., "The Seductive Allure of Neuroscience Explanations"; Weisberg, Taylor, and Hopkins, "Deconstructing the Seductive Allure of Neuroscience Explanations."

26. Remmel, Glenn, and Cox, "Biological Evidence regarding Psychopathy Does Not Affect Mock Jury Sentencing."

27. Scurich and Shniderman, "The Selective Allure of Neuroscientific Explanations," 4.

28. Nelson, *The Social Life of DNA*; Roth and Ivemark, "Genetic Options"; Shim, Alam, and Aouizerat, "Knowing Something versus Feeling Different." See also Novas and Rose, "Genetic Risk and the Birth of the Somatic Individual."

29. Alač, "Digital Scientific Visuals as Fields for Interaction," 66.

30. This again demonstrates the role of boundary objects in the neuroscience of violence. And, similar to the fluid use of diagnostic tools examined in Chapter 2, this is a larger critique of the tools of neuropsychological and the mind and brain sciences more generally. See Rijcke and Beaulieu, "Networked Neuroscience."

31. Roskies, "Neuroimaging and Inferential Distance."

32. Rijcke and Beaulieu, "Networked Neuroscience," 131.

33. My point here is not to make a redundant argument about the function of the gaze, but to use Foucault's powerful conception of medical authority as a starting point to trace the impacts of the practice of visualization in the neuroscience of violence. For more on the "gaze" in biocriminology or the biology of violence, see Rose, "'Screen and Intervene'"; Walby and Carrier, "The Rise of Biocriminology"; Becker, "The Criminologists' Gaze at the Underworld."

34. Foucault, *The Birth of the Clinic*.

35. Lupton, "Foucault and the Medicalisation Critique," 99 (emphasis added).

36. Foucault, *The Birth of the Clinic*.

37. Lynch, "Representation in Formation," 325.

38. Niehoff, *The Biology of Violence*.

39. Interview, Dr. Moore, 1/24/13.

40. Poldrack, "Can Cognitive Processes Be Inferred from Neuroimaging Data?," 59.

41. Poldrack, *The New Mind Readers*.

42. Aguirre, "Functional Imaging in Behavioral Neurology and Cognitive Neuropsychology."

43. At least eight studies applied CT technologies to study violence during the 1980s. However, more than half of these studies found no significant difference between the subject groups. See Raine, *The Psychopathology of Crime*.

44. Volkow and Tancredi, "Neural Substrates of Violent Behaviour."

45. Raine, Buchsbaum et al., "Selective Reductions in Prefrontal Glucose Metabolism in Murderers"; Raine, Buchsbaum, and Lacasse, "Brain Abnormalities in Murderers Indicated by Positron Emission Tomography"; Raine et al., "Prefrontal Glucose Deficits in Murderers Lacking Psychosocial Deprivation"; Raine et al., "Reduced Prefrontal and Increased Subcortical Brain Functioning Assessed Using Positron Emission Tomography in Predatory and Affective Murderers."

46. Raichle, "A Brief History of Human Brain Mapping."

47. Rosvold et al., "A Continuous Performance Test of Brain Damage"; Nuechterlein, Parasuraman, and Jiang, "Visual Sustained Attention"; Buchsbaum et al., "Glucose Metabolic Rate in Normals and Schizophrenics during the Continuous Performance Test Assessed by Positron Emission Tomography"; Riccio et al., "The Continuous Performance Test." The CPT dates to early twentieth-century EEG imaging research on brain damage (Rosvold et al. 1956). During the scan, participants are asked to watch a monitor that will briefly display a set of stimuli at a predetermined rate, and each time the participant recognizes the stimulus they are told to acknowledge it by pressing a button (Nuechterlein, Parasuraman, and Jiang, "Visual Sustained Attention").

48. Raine, Buchsbaum, and Lacasse, "Brain Abnormalities in Murderers Indicated by Positron Emission Tomography."

49. Raine, Buchsbaum, and Lacasse.

50. Raine, Buchsbaum et al., "Selective Reductions in Prefrontal Glucose Metabolism in Murderers," 372.

51. Latour and Woolgar, *Laboratory Life*; Knorr-Cetina, *Epistemic Cultures*.

52. Hacking, "Degeneracy, Criminal Behavior, and Looping."

53. Interview, Dr. Garrett, 11/14/11.

54. Adams, "How to Spot a Murderer's Brain"; Raine, *The Anatomy of Violence*.

55. Gould, *The Mismeasure of Man*.

56. Lewis et al., "The Mismeasure of Science."

57. See Lewis et al., 1.

58. Gould, *The Mismeasure of Man*, 12.

59. Aguirre, "Functional Imaging in Behavioral Neurology and Cognitive Neuropsychology"; Meyer-Lindenberg, "From Maps to Mechanisms through Neuroimaging of Schizophrenia."

60. Prior to the Raine et al. 2000 article, there were a few studies that used MRI. However, these studies either combined this technology with others like CT or used the technology to study violence within populations diagnosed with personality disorders that were outside the scope of this study (i.e., schizophrenia). See Bassarath, "Neuroimaging Studies of Antisocial Behaviour."

61. Gray matter is recognized anatomically as brain areas where neuronal signaling originates. It is what defines higher-level executive functioning, and thereby the source of cognitions and actions, or essentially what makes us human.

62. Raine et al., "Reduced Prefrontal Gray Matter Volume and Reduced Autonomic Activity in Antisocial Personality Disorder," 125 (emphasis added).

63. Damasio et al., "The Return of Phineas Gage," 1102.

64. Harlow, "Recovery from the Passage of an Iron Bar through the Head (Originally Published 1868)," 277.

65. Damasio et al., "The Return of Phineas Gage."

66. Damasio, *Descartes' Error*.

67. Raine, *The Anatomy of Violence*.

68. Kiehl, *The Psychopath Whisperer*, 170 (emphasis in original). See also *The Science of Evil*, 82, in which Baron-Cohen writes that "Gage suffered [brain] damage to his entire [orbitofrontal cortex] and [ventral medial prefrontal cortex] and began showing signs of callous, rude, irreverent, and disinhibited behavior." Similarly, in Glenn and Raine's *Psychopathy: An Introduction*, 90, they state that "Gage did not have deficits in intelligence and reasoning likely because the dorsolateral region of the [prefrontal cortex] remained intact."

69. Becker, "New Monsters on the Block?," 277.

70. Interview, Dr. Lewis, 11/7/11.

71. Rose and Abi-Rached, *Neuro*, 81.

72. Foucault, *The Birth of the Clinic*, 169 (emphasis in original).

73. Aguirre, "Functional Imaging in Behavioral Neurology and Cognitive Neuropsychology." This description also comes from my notes on Geoffrey Aguirre's lecture on fMRI during my participation in the University of Pennsylvania's Center for Neuroscience Neuroscience Boot Camp, August 2013.

74. Interview, Dr. Smith, 5/7/12.

75. Interview, Dr. Smith, 5/7/12.

76. Interview, Dr. Hollowell, 10/29/11.

77. Barrett et al., "The Experience of Emotion."

78. Lisa Barrett and colleagues make it clear that "at present, it is not possible to causally reduce these experiences to neurobiological processes and explain how neural activity instantiates specific emotional contents (or any conscious contents for that matter)" (381). Instead they have suggested that the link between

the brain and emotions be described as a neural reference space—what they see as "a preliminary sketch of the brain areas that are active during experiences of emotion (i.e., a neural reference space for mental representations of emotion)."

79. Davidson, Putnam, and Larson, "Dysfunction in the Neural Circuitry of Emotion Regulation," 591.

80. Herpertz et al., "Emotional Processing in Male Adolescents with Childhood-Onset Conduct Disorder"; Decety et al., "Atypical Empathic Responses in Adolescents with Aggressive Conduct Disorder"; see also Coccaro et al., "Amygdala and Orbitofrontal Reactivity to Social Threat in Individuals with Impulsive Aggression."

81. Blair, "Too Much of a Good Thing"; Coccaro et al., "Amygdala and Orbitofrontal Reactivity to Social Threat in Individuals with Impulsive Aggression."

82. Pickersgill, "Ordering Disorder," 71. See also Star, *Regions of the Mind*.

83. Abend, "What Are Neural Correlates Neural Correlates Of?"

84. Dumit, "How (Not) to Do Things with Brain Images"; Pickersgill, "Between Soma and Society."

85. Interview, Dr. Jones, 4/23/12.

86. Interview, Dr. Jones, 4/23/12.

87. Sterzer et al., "Abnormal Neural Responses to Emotional Visual Stimuli in Adolescents with Conduct Disorder."

88. The Sterzer et al. study had 27 participants, 13 in the target group and 14 in the control group.

89. Sterzer et al., "Abnormal Neural Responses to Emotional Visual Stimuli in Adolescents with Conduct Disorder," 12.

90. Faigman, Monahan, and Slobogin, "Group to Individual (G2i) Inference in Scientific Expert Testimony."

91. Faigman, Monahan, and Slobogin.

92. Siever, "Neurobiology of Aggression and Violence," 429.

93. Siever, 429.

94. Pietrini et al., "Neural Correlates of Imaginal Aggressive Behavior Assessed by Positron Emission Tomography in Healthy Subjects." This study was done in 2000 using PET imaging, but it is important because it was one of the first to focus on neurobiological factors of violence in healthy subjects. The authors' goal was to demonstrate the modulating role of the orbitofrontal cortex (OFC) on aggressive behavior. The OFC has been associated with regulating emotion, including regulating punishment- and reward-related behavior, and impulsive drives.

95. Pietrini et al., 1773. Each scenario pertained to a specific test: the first was cognitive restraint, the second was physical restraint, and the third was unre-

strained aggression. The authors noted: "A standard description of each scenario was read to the subjects immediately before the radioisotope injection; subjects were instructed to keep their eyes closed, to listen carefully to the script, and to focus on the evoked situation until they were told to stop. Each imagined condition lasted for approximately 100 seconds. . . . Before the scan, subjects were instructed that they would have to evoke imagined situations during the study, but to maintain novelty, no details about the nature of the scenarios were provided."

96. Joyce, "Neuroimaging Production in Clinical Practice."

97. Pietrini et al., "Neural Correlates of Imaginal Aggressive Behavior Assessed by Positron Emission Tomography in Healthy Subjects," 1779.

98. Canguilhem, *The Normal and the Pathological*, 243.

99. Canguilhem, *The Normal and the Pathological*; Durkheim, *The Division of Labor in Society*.

CHAPTER 4

1. Lindesmith and Levin, "The Lombrosian Myth in Criminology"; see also Rafter, *The Criminal Brain*.

2. To be clear, Lombroso too viewed factors such as race and gender as biological, and important to his theory of the born criminal—which was, in part, the reason he took notice of them in his theories. See Rafter, *The Criminal Brain*.

3. Lindesmith and Levin, "The Lombrosian Myth in Criminology," 666–67n21.

4. Lindesmith and Levin, 666–67n21.

5. Fink, *Causes of Crime*, 251 (emphasis added).

6. Eysenck, *Crime and Personality*.

7. Mark, "Social and Ethical Issues," 1.

8. Interview, Dr. Fitzpatrick, 1/14/12 (emphasis added).

9. Lemke, *Biopolitics*, 19.

10. Jacobs et al., "Aggressive Behavior, Mental Sub-Normality and the XYY Male."

11. Jeffery, "Criminology as an Interdisciplinary Behavioral Science."

12. In addition to the XYY karyotype analysis, Hannell underwent both a general intelligence evaluation, which showed a below-average intelligence and, interestingly, an electroencephalogram (EEG) exam, which showed abnormal activity in the right temporal lobe of the brain—this would not be the last time that brain technologies would be used in conjunction with genetic approaches to violent behavior.

13. Bartholomew and Sutherland, "A Defence of Insanity and the Extra Y Chromosome."

14. *New York Times,* "Extra Chromosome Brings an Acquittal on Murder Charge," October 10, 1968, 94.

15. Stock, "The XYY and the Criminal," *New York Times,* October 20, 1968.

16. Royce, *The XYY Man.*

17. Beckwith, "The Persistent Influence of Failed Scientific Ideas"; Witkin et al., "Criminality in XYY and XXY Men."

18. Nelkin and Swazey, "Science and Social Control"; Beckwith, "The Persistent Influence of Failed Scientific Ideas."

19. *People v. Tanner,* 13 *Cal. App. 3d* 596. Also cited in *People v. Yukl,* 83 Misc. 2d 364 (N.Y. Misc. 1975).

20. However—and despite such clear methodological problems and theoretical inaccuracies—as recently as 2012 a team of researchers in Denmark tried again to establish a link between XYY and crime. See Stochholm et al., "Criminality in Men with Klinefelter's Syndrome and XYY Syndrome." Nevertheless, when the researchers adjusted for social factors like education and poverty, this variance between the groups decreased and was no longer statistically significant, underscoring the point of critics that social/environmental factors often explain much more of the variance in violence than biological markers do.

21. Richardson, *Sex Itself,* 101.

22. Carey and Gottesman, "Genetics and Antisocial Behavior," 88, 89.

23. Messerschmidt, *Crime as Structured Action.*

24. Connell, *Masculinities;* Messerschmidt, *Masculinities and Crime.*

25. Messerschmidt, *Masculinities and Crime,* 85.

26. This more-complex view of the gender-violence dynamic recognizes that such behaviors discursively reconstitute and empower the seemingly natural fact that men are inherently more powerful and aggressive, and productively enact and preserve these ideas of social order and privilege through complexly intersected social locations of gender, race, sexuality, class, and ableism. For further reading, see Connell and Messerschmidt, "Hegemonic Masculinity"; Jordan-Young and Karkazis, *Testosterone.*

27. Jordan-Young and Karkazis, *Testosterone.*

28. Jordan-Young and Karkazis, *Testosterone,* 77–82.

29. Jordan-Young and Karkazis, *Testosterone.*

30. Mednick and Volavka, "Biology and Crime."

31. Mednick and Volavka.

32. Raine, *The Psychopathology of Crime.*

33. Mednick, Gabrielli, and Hutchings, "Genetic Influences in Criminal Convictions," 893.

34. Panofsky, *Misbehaving Science.*

35. Rose, *The Politics of Life Itself.*

36. Panofsky, *Misbehaving Science.*

37. Morell, "Evidence Found for a Possible 'Aggression Gene.'"

38. MAOA is located on the X chromosome; thus it was transmitted from mother to son.

39. Brunner et al., "Abnormal Behavior Associated with a Point Mutation in the Structural Gene for Monoamine Oxidase A."

40. Brunner, "Monoamine Oxidase and Behaviour," 432.

41. Cases et al., "Aggressive Behavior and Altered Amounts of Brain Serotonin and Norepinephrine in Mice Lacking MAOA"; Shih and Chen, "MAO-A and -B Gene Knock-out Mice Exhibit Distinctly Different Behavior."

42. Meyer-Lindenberg et al., "Neural Mechanisms of Genetic Risk for Impulsivity and Violence in Humans."

43. Caspi et al., "Role of Genotype in the Cycle of Violence in Maltreated Children."

44. Haberstick et al., "Monoamine Oxidase A (MAOA) and Antisocial Behaviors in the Presence of Childhood and Adolescent Maltreatment"; Ficks and Waldman, "Candidate Genes for Aggression and Antisocial Behavior"; Byrd and Manuck, "MAOA, Childhood Maltreatment, and Antisocial Behavior"; Goldman and Rosser, "MAOA-Environment Interactions."

45. Many of the most egregious (mis)uses of this research come out of criminology. Criminological interpretations of genetics have also contributed widely to the racial controversy with MAOA. See Larregue and Rollins, "Biosocial Criminology and the Mismeasure of Race"; Larregue, *Héréditaire.*

46. Gibbons, "Tracking the Evolutionary History of a 'Warrior' Gene."

47. Merriman and Cameron, "Risk-Taking."

48. Lea and Chambers, "Monoamine Oxidase, Addiction, and the 'Warrior' Gene Hypothesis."

49. Lea and Chambers, 3–4 (emphasis added).

50. Gillett and Tamatea, "The Warrior Gene," 50–51.

51. Young and Balaban, "Aggression, Biology, and Context," 194.

52. Buckholtz and Meyer-Lindenberg, "MAOA and the Bioprediction of Antisocial Behavior," 141.

53. Vassos, Collier, and Fazel, "Systematic Meta-Analyses and Field Synopsis of Genetic Association Studies of Violence and Aggression," 474.

54. Buckholtz and Meyer-Lindenberg, "MAOA and the Bioprediction of Antisocial Behavior."

55. Jeffery, "Criminology as an Interdisciplinary Behavioral Science," 157.

56. Carrier and Walby, "Ptolemizing Lombroso."

57. Interview, Dr. Hollowell, 10/29/11.

58. Raine et al., "Biosocial Bases of Violence," 2.

59. See Platt and Takagi, "Biosocial Criminology"; see also Carrier and Walby, "Ptolemizing Lombroso."

60. There has been, however, epigenetic research on violence that would get closer to this intersectional view. Epigenetics refers to the opposite, the way environments influence the expression of biological factors. This is not a matter of which gene, but a question of if and why gene expression manifests under certain environmental conditions. See Landecker and Panofsky, "From Social Structure to Gene Regulation, and Back." However, it still can be argued that even in the more advanced epigenetic claim, there still is a limited way in which we can understand a variable as a truly biosocial one, a uniquely integrated "new" type of variable

61. Interview, Dr. Hollowell, 10/29/11.

62. Interview, Dr. Hollowell, 10/29/11.

63. See: Caspi et al., "Role of Genotype in the Cycle of Violence in Maltreated Children"; Craig, "The Role of Monoamine Oxidase A, MAOA, in the Aetiology of Antisocial Behaviour."

64. Buckholtz and Meyer-Lindenberg, "Gene-Brain Associations: The Example of MAOA," 275.]

65. Interview, Dr. Hollowell, 10/29/11.

66. Niehoff, *The Biology of Violence*, 30.

67. Interview, Dr. Jones, 4/23/12.

68. Viding and McCrory, "Genetic Biomarker Research of Callous-Unemotional Traits in Children," 163.

69. Lappé, "The Maternal Body as Environment in Autism Science."

70. Raine, "Biosocial Studies of Antisocial and Violent Behavior in Children and Adults: A Review."

71. Raine, "From Genes to Brain to Antisocial Behavior."

72. Raine, "Biosocial Studies of Antisocial and Violent Behavior in Children and Adults."

73. Interview, Dr. Jones, 4/23/12.

74. Interview, Dr. Fitzpatrick, 1/14/12.

75. Strauss, *Continual Permutations of Action*; Blumer, *Symbolic Interactionism*.

76. Raine et al., "Biosocial Bases of Violence," 2.

77. DiLalla and Gottesman, "Biological and Genetic Contributors to Violence," 125.

78. Umhau et al., "The Physician's Unique Role in Preventing Violence."

79. Umhau et al., 1.

80. Timmermans, "Matching Genotype and Phenotype," 137.

81. Timmermans, 137.

82. Panofsky, *Misbehaving Science*, 166.

83. Panofsky, 166.

CHAPTER 5

1. Omi and Winant, *Racial Formation in the United States*, 56. Sociologists Michael Omi and Howard Winant define racial projects as "simultaneously an interpretation, representation, or explanation of racial dynamics, and an effort to reorganize and redistribute resources along particular racial lines."

2. Lombroso, *Criminal Man*, 91.

3. Simon, "Positively Punitive." Simon notes that the influence of Lombroso lives on today through penal policies such as the death penalty, preventive detention, sexual violent predator civil commitment laws, renewed interest in criminal rehabilitation, and indeterminate sentencing patterns.

4. To be clear, the "born criminal" thesis was a contentious and controversial idea within German biocriminology, and genetic determinism and scientist racism did not overpower other criminological knowledges. That is, there was "a certain amount of 'normal science' that continued with the Nazi regime" (Wetzell, "Criminology in Weimar and Nazi Germany," 423). This is not to absolve the program of its influence on racial sterilization or scientific racism at this time, but it does better contextualize how today's more nuanced and less obvious ways of employing racial politics can easily be reconstituted through scientific knowledge.

5. Barkan, *The Retreat of Scientific Racism*; Reardon, *Race to the Finish*; Stepan, *The Idea of Race in Science*; Yudell, *Race Unmasked*.

6. It should be noted that IQ is still used as a variable in criminology, and that its more biologized understandings also still have life in certain factions of today's biosocial criminology. See Larregue and Rollins, "Biosocial Criminology and the Mismeasure of Race"; Carrier and Walby, "Ptolemizing Lombroso."

7. Eysenck, *Race, Intelligence, and Education*.

8. Eysenck, *Race, Intelligence, and Education*, 11.

9. Valenstein, *The Psychosurgery Debate*.

10. Valenstein, 12.

11. Mark, Sweet, and Ervin, "Role of Brain Disease in Riots and Urban Violence," 1967, 895.

12. Pollack, "Role of Brain Disease in Riots and Urban Violence."

13. Mark, Sweet, and Ervin, "Role of Brain Disease in Riots and Urban Violence," 1968, 368 (emphasis in original).

14. Pollack, "Role of Brain Disease in Riots and Urban Violence."

15. Quoted in Mason, "New Threat to Blacks," 63–64 (emphasis in original).

16. Baldwin, "The Negro and the American Promise."

17. "Ebony Magazine, Letters to the Editor—Brain Surgery," 9–10.

18. Metzl, *The Protest Psychosis*. Metzl demonstrates that Detroit law enforcement and mental health officials worked together to respond to the city's growing civil unrest. As a result, a disproportionate number of African American men involved in the civil rights movement and/or protest demonstrations were arrested and sent to mental health facilities. Psychiatrists treating these "patients" viewed their supposed "aggressive" and/or "violent" behavioral patterns as indicative of a mental illness, and as a result these men were officially diagnosed as schizophrenic.

19. "Ebony Magazine, Letters to the Editor—Psychosurgery." The Report and Recommendation for Psychosurgery was published in 1977 by the National Commission for the Protection of Human Subjects of Biomedical and Behavioral Research.

20. Mark, "Social and Ethical Issues."

21. Ervin, "Violence and Brain Disease."

22. Ervin, 1464.

23. Congressional hearings were conducted in response to the proposed joint funding of the center by the National Institutes of Health and the Department of Justice. On the public responses and legal challenges to the center, see Marsh and Katz, *Biology, Crime and Ethics*; Moran, "Medicine and Crime"; Alondra Nelson, *Body and Soul*; National Commission for the Protection of Human Subjects of Biomedical and Behavioral Research, "Psychosurgery."

24. Mark, "Social and Ethical Issues," 249 (emphasis added).

25. Hatch, *Blood Sugar*. Hatch makes a similar argument concerning metabolic syndrome, contending that biomedical practices seem detached from racial meaning, but in fact race is now being repacked at the molecular level, and therefore plays a power role in making sense of biomedical knowledges. See also Roberts, *Fatal Invention*.

26. Bonilla-Silva, *Racism without Racists*; Bonilla-Silva, "Rethinking Racism"; Brown et al., *Whitewashing Race*; Obasogie, *Blinded by Sight*.

27. Bonilla-Silva, "Rethinking Racism"; Bobo, Kluegel, and Smith, "Laissez-Faire Racism"; Balibar, "Is There a 'Neo-Racism'"; Omi and Winant, *Racial Formation in the United States*.

28. Bonilla-Silva, *Racism without Racists*.

29. Fishbein, *Biobehavioral Perspectives on Criminology*, 94 (emphasis in original). Importantly, Fishbein is a former student of criminologist Clarence

R. Jeffery, one of the first scholars to advocate a "biosocial criminology. (See Jeffrey, "Criminology as an Interdisciplinary Behavioral Science.")

30. M'charek, Schramm, and Skinner, "Technologies of Belonging."

31. M'charek, Schramm, and Skinner, 459.

32. Interview, Dr. Moore, 1/24/13.

33. Dumit, *Picturing Personhood*, 62–63. PET (positron emission technology) imaging.

34. Epstein, *Inclusion*.

35. Zuberi, *Thicker Than Blood*; see also Zuberi and Bonilla-Silva, *White Logic, White Methods*.

36. Roberts, *Fatal Invention*.

37. Interview, Dr. Smith, 5/7/12.

38. Bonilla-Silva, *Racism without Racists*; Brown et al., *Whitewashing Race*.

39. Goldberg, *The Threat of Race*, 8–9.

40. Dr. Smith, Interview, 5/7/12.

41. Dr. McKinney, Interview, 4/11/12.

42. Unlike the genetic sciences, the neurosciences have produced no known work examining the use of race,, hence this institutionalized practice of talking about race in privacy may be endemic to neuroscience research on social behaviors in general, and not just limited to research on violence.

43. Interview, Dr. Jones, 4/23/12 (emphasis added).

44. Omi and Winant, *Racial Formation in the United States*; Bonilla-Silva, "Rethinking Racism."

45. Bonilla-Silva, "Rethinking Racism"; Goldberg, *The Racial State*; Hall, "Who Needs Identity?"; Omi and Winant, *Racial Formation in the United States*.

46. Dr. Lewis, Interview, 11/7/11.

47. Omi and Winant, *Racial Formation in the United States*.

48. Shim, *Heart-Sick*, 88–98.

49. Shim, 108.

50. Barkan, *The Retreat of Scientific Racism*; Feagin, *Systemic Racism*; Gilroy, *There Ain't No Black in the Union Jack*.

51. Wade, *Race and Ethnicity in Latin America*, 19.

52. Muhammad, *The Condemnation of Blackness*.

53. Pretus et al., "Neural and Behavioral Correlates of Sacred Values and Vulnerability to Violent Extremism"; Hamid et al., "Neuroimaging 'Will to Fight' for Sacred Values."

54. Hamid, "What I Learned from Scanning the Brains of Potential Terrorists."

55. Pretus et al., "Neural and Behavioral Correlates of Sacred Values and Vulnerability to Violent Extremism."

56. Silva, *Brown Threat*, 29.

57. Silva, *Brown Threat*, 29–30 (emphasis in original).

58. Du Bois, *Souls of Black Folk*, 7

59. Armenta, "Racializing Crimmigration"; Browne, *Dark Matters*; Pinder-hughes, *Race in the Hood*; Rios, *Punished*; Silva, *Brown Threat*; Wacquant, "From Slavery to Mass Incarceration."

60. Hyde et al., "Dissecting the Role of Amygdala Reactivity in Antisocial Behavior in a Sample of Young, Low-Income, Urban Men," 529.

61. Tomlinson et al., "Neighborhood Poverty Predicts Altered Neural and Behavioral Response Inhibition," 7.

62. For an overview of the neuroimaging research on racial recognition and racial bias, see Kubota, Banaji, and Phelps, "The Neuroscience of Race." Roberts and Rollins, "Why Sociology Matters to Race and Biosocial Science" provides a sociological overview of this research and a critique of its potential social impacts. Jonathan Kahn's book *Race on the Brain* provides an extensive critique of the use of implicit racial bias neuroscience research in law.

63. Kubota, Banaji, and Phelps, "The Neuroscience of Race."

64. Hawkins, *Ethnicity, Race, and Crime*, 41 (emphasis in original).

65. Shim, "Bio-Power and Racial, Class, and Gender Formation in Biomedical Knowledge Production"; Shim, *Heart-Sick*.

66. Hall, "Who Needs Identity?"

67. Duster, "Explaining Differential Trust," 3.

68. Duster, "Explaining Differential Trust," 3; see also Ann Morning, *The Nature of Race*, 153.

69. Benjamin, "Innovating Inequity."

70. The term "trans-science" was coined by nuclear physicist Alvin Weinberg, who defined it as "questions of fact [that] can be stated in the language of science, [but] they are unanswerable by science; they transcend science"; see Weinberg, "Science and Trans-Science," 209. More recently, Alondra Nelson, *The Social Life of DNA*, 163–66, has applied the "trans-scientific" critique to the unsettled debates around race and genetics, that are now prominently displayed in the increasing use of direct-to-consumer ancestry testing. Nelson persuasively argues that genetic science is unable to grapple with and/or adjudicate the deeply embedded ethical, metaphysical, and moral questions about identity, power, and justice.

CHAPTER 6

1. Moran, "Medicine and Crime," 222.

2. Dick, *Selected Stories of Philip K. Dick*, 225.

3. Adams, Murphy, and Clarke, "Anticipation."

4. Interview, Dr. Moore, 1/24/13.

5. Interview, Dr. Lewis, 11/7/11.

6. Marcus, *Technoscientific Imaginaries*, 4.

7. Thompson, *Making Parents*; Rubin, "Therapeutic Promise in the Discourse of Human Embryonic Stem Cell Research."

8. Thompson, *Making Parents*; Rajan, *Biocapital*. See also Clarke et al., *Biomedicalization*.

9. Thompson, *Making Parents*, 255–58. Similarly, anthropologist Kaushik Sunder Rajan considers the notion of "promissory biocapital." Drawing a distinction between "therapeutic realization" and "commercial realization" of capital, Rajan argues that the former goes beyond commercial value—the seamless reproduction of things that already exist. Instead, therapeutic value helps to remake surplus value, now understood through a "creative potential" that rearticulates value and meaning for scientific facts. Rajan, *Biocapital*, 113–15.

10. Rubin, "Therapeutic Promise in the Discourse of Human Embryonic Stem Cell Research."

11. Rose, "'Screen and Intervene.'"

12. Rose, 96.

13. Rose, 80. Rose describes the emergence of the susceptible individual as the bringing together of two forms of risk—to others and to self. He notes that "screen and intervene" operates in three important ways: (1) making neurobiology central to understanding conduct for the normal and pathological, (2) identifying risk presymptomatically or asymptomatically, and (3) practicing pre-caution, in which prevention is best understood as intervention during earliest stages of life possible."

14. Interview, Dr. Lewis, 11/7/11.

15. Interview, Dr. Jones, 4/23/12.

16. Interview, Dr. Jones, 4/23/12.

17. Interview, Dr. Hollowell.

18. Dumit, *Picturing Personhood*, 7. The "objective-self" refers to the often taken-for-granted ways we come to receive and "know" how neuroscientifically produced brain facts matter for our bodies and selves.

19. Dumit, 166.

20. Tolwinski, "Fraught Claims at the Intersection of Biology and Sociality," reached a similar conclusion through an examination of the management of controversy in the neuroscience of poverty.

21. Raine et al., "Early Educational and Health Enrichment at Age 3–5 Years Is Associated with Increased Autonomic and Central Nervous System Arousal and Orienting at Age 11 Years"; see also Glenn and Raine, "Neurocriminology."

22. Kirkpatrick, McIntyre, and Potestio, "Child Hunger and Long-Term Adverse Consequences for Health."

23. Glenn and Raine, "Neurocriminology."

24. Kirby et al., "A Double-Blind, Placebo-Controlled Study Investigating the Effects of Omega-3 Supplementation in Children Aged 8–10 Years from a Mainstream School Population"; Bloch and Qawasmi, "Omega-3 Fatty Acid Supplementation for the Treatment of Children with Attention-Deficit/Hyperactivity Disorder Symptomatology."

25. Zaalberg et al., "Effects of Nutritional Supplements on Aggression, Rule-Breaking, and Psychopathology among Young Adult Prisoners."

26. Interview, Dr. Garrett, 11/14/11.

27. Moffitt, "Adolescence-Limited and Life-Course-Persistent Antisocial Behavior."

28. Sampson and Laub, "A Life-Course View of the Development of Crime," 40. This argument is in response to the primacy given to critical periods of development in Moffitt's life-course perspective. Sampson and Laub argue that criminal offending and desistance are not unique to specific developmental trajectories, but common to all offenders (i.e., both life-course and adolescent limited). Their argument "underscores how people construct their lives within the context of ongoing constraints. From this view, trajectories are interpreted not from a lens of unfolding inevitability but rather continuous social reproduction" (14).

29. The Mauritius Child Health Project was started in the 1970s by psychologist Peter Venables (Raine's mentor), geneticist Sarnoff Mednick, and Fini Schulsinger. It has continued with the support of the Mauritian government, as well as researcher funding from NIH and other agencies. See Raine et al., "Cohort Profile."

30. Raine et al., "Early Educational and Health Enrichment at Age 3–5 Years Is Associated with Increased Autonomic and Central Nervous System Arousal and Orienting at Age 11 Years," 256.

31. Pinderhughes, *Changing Landscapes of Violence through Social and Physical Interventions*; Pinderhughes, Davis, and Williams, "Adverse Community Experiences and Resilience."

32. Pitts-Taylor, *The Brain's Body*.

33. Landecker, "Food as Exposure."

34. There does exist robust evidence illustrating a connection between overall nutritional health and children's social well-being and their ability to concentrate and learn in school;similarly, there is also evidence showing a connection between "food deserts" in the United States and poorer health outcomes in general. Thus, I do not doubt that the value of good nutrition may lead to positive

psychological, developmental, and social performance and outcomes. Instead, I am concerned about the way in which the violent brain is attached to this ideal. See Walker, Keane, and Burke, "Disparities and Access to Healthy Food in the United States"; Lewis et al., "African Americans' Access to Healthy Food Options in South Los Angeles Restaurants."

35. Viding and McCrory, "Genetic Biomarker Research of Callous-Unemotional Traits in Children."

36. NIH, "Gene Therapy."

37. Viding and McCrory, "Genetic Biomarker Research of Callous-Unemotional Traits in Children."

38. Interview, Dr. Garrett, 11/14/11.

39. Novas and Rose, "Genetic Risk and the Birth of the Somatic Individual," 502.

40. See Arribas-Ayllon, Sarangi, and Clarke, "The Micropolitics of Responsibility vis-à-vis Autonomy"; Etchegary et al., "Decision-Making about Inherited Cancer Risk."

41. Interview, Dr. Moore, 1/24/13.

42. Broer and Pickersgill, "Targeting Brains, Producing Responsibilities," 57.

43. Pitts-Taylor, "Neurobiologically Poor?"; also see Tolwinski, "Fraught Claims at the Intersection of Biology and Sociality."

44. Tolwinski, "Fraught Claims at the Intersection of Biology and Sociality."

45. Pitts-Taylor, *The Brain's Body*, 41.

46. Roberts, *Killing the Black Body*.

47. Walsh, "Youth Justice and Neuroscience."

48. Walsh, "Youth Justice and Neuroscience."

49. Poldrack et al., "Predicting Violent Behavior."

50. Interview, Dr. McKinney, 4/11/12.

51. Interview, Dr. Jones, 4/23/12.

52. Haynes and Rees, "Decoding Mental States from Brain Activity in Humans," 523.

53. Scheinost et al., "Ten Simple Rules for Predictive Modeling of Individual Differences in Neuroimaging"; Falk, Berkman, and Lieberman, "From Neural Responses to Population Behavior"; Berkman and Falk, "Beyond Brain Mapping."

54. Jones and Shen, "Law and Neuroscience in the United States."

55. Greely and Farahany, "Neuroscience and the Criminal Justice System," 453; see also Farahany, "Neuroscience and Behavioral Genetics in US Criminal Law."

56. Dumit, "How (Not) to Do Things with Brain Images."

57. Dumit, "How (Not) to Do Things with Brain Images."

58. Nadelhoffer and Sinnott-Armstrong, "Neurolaw and Neuroprediction."

59. Interview, Dr. McKinney, 4/11/12.

60. Dumit, *Picturing Personhood*.

61. Interview, Dr. Fitzpatrick, 4/23/12.

62. Aharoni et al., "Neuroprediction of Future Rearrest." The study covered a four-year period and included both violent and nonviolent crimes; thus the findings should be interpreted with caution in regard to violence.

63. For critiques of Kiehl's neuroprediction, see Poldrack et al., "Predicting Violent Behavior."

64. Kiehl et al., "Age of Gray Matters," 822.

65. Alexander, *The New Jim Crow*; Muhammad, *The Condemnation of Blackness*; Wacquant, *Punishing the Poor*; Roberts, *Killing the Black Body*; Pager, "The Mark of a Criminal Record"; Eubanks, *Automating Inequality*; Rios, *Punished*.

66. Interview, Dr. Holmes, 10/4/12.

67. Raine, *The Anatomy of Violence*.

68. Raine (in a personal conversation in Spring 2017) expressed regret about the inclusion of the fictional predictive program, which he felt took away from the book's overall message about the significance of neurobiological risk for violence.

69. Raine, *The Anatomy of Violence*, 354.

70. Familial DNA matches are *partial* matches established between DNA found at a crime scene and existing DNA profiles in criminal databases. See Greely et al., "Family Ties," for an overview. For a critical legal viewpoint, see Murphy, "Familial DNA Searches."

71. Selk, "The Ingenious and 'Dystopian' DNA Technique Police Used to Hunt the 'Golden State Killer' Suspect."

72. Erlich et al., "Identity Inference of Genomic Data Using Long-Range Familial Searches."

73. Murphy, "Familial DNA Searches."

74. Duster, "Behavioral Genetics and the Link between Crime, Violence, and Race"; Rollins, "Risky Bodies."

75. Bliss, *Social by Nature*; as an example, see Conley and Fletcher, *The Genome Factor*.

76. Heinemann, Lemke, and Prainsack, "Risky Profiles"; Lee and Voigt, "DNA Testing for Family Reunification and the Limits of Biological Truth."

77. Raine, *The Anatomy of Violence*, 357.

78. The Health Insurance Portability and Accountability Act (HIPAA) was implemented in 1996 to establish how medical information is stored and the safeguards put in place to protect individuals' privacy. (See hhs.gov/hipaa/for-professionals/privacy/index.html.)

79. Pickersgill, "The Co-Production of Science, Ethics, and Emotion."

CHAPTER 7

1. Beckwith, "The Persistent Influence of Failed Scientific Ideas."

2. Rose and Abi-Rached, *Neuro*, 162.

3. Pitts-Taylor, *The Brain's Body*; Pickersgill, "The Social Life of the Brain."

4. De Vos, "What Is Critique in the Era of the Neurosciences?," 25.

5. Dumit, *Picturing Personhood*, 177.

6. Rose ("'Screen and Intervene,'" 97) does not explicitly make this relational link, but he does push for an understanding of "screen and intervene" as distinct from "discipline and punish."

7. Pickersgill, "The Co-Production of Science, Ethics, and Emotion."

8. See Foucault, *Discipline and Punish*; Foucault, *Security, Territory, Population*.

9. Foucault, *Security, Territory, Population*.

10. Foucault, *Security, Territory, Population*, 87.

11. Lemke, *Biopolitics*, 47.

12. Canguilhem, *The Normal and the Pathological*, 247.

13. Wacquant, *Punishing the Poor*.

14. Field notes, Neuroscience Bootcamp (August 2013), UC Hastings Law and Neuro Conference.

15. Alexander, *The New Jim Crow*, 188.

16. Dumit, "The Fragile Unity of Neuroscience."

17. Wacquant, *Punishing the Poor*.

18. Lemke, *Biopolitics*, 31.

19. Goldberg, *The Threat of Race*, 334.

20. Fassin (*Life*) and Weheliye (*Habeas Viscus*) both provide excellent critiques of the ability of biopolitical theories to address racial inequality. See also Roberts, "Law, Race, and Biotechnology"; Reardon, "The Democratic, Anti-Racist Genome?"

21. Star, *Regions of the Mind*, 16.

22. Both Bonilla-Silva and Obasogie remind us that color-blind logics are made real through social discourse and practices. I'm arguing that social dynamics can also be built into scientific technologies, and are even more salient in biological discourses, which are always part of "racializing assemblages," which produce racial categories but also the relational pathways through which they are articulated and experienced. Bonilla-Silva, *Racism without Racists*; Obasogie, *Blinded by Sight*. See also Weheliye, *Habeas Viscus*.

23. Fassin, *Life*, 125.

24. Fassin (*Life*, 124–25) argues that "the reality of unequal lives is not a new discovery made by social scientists: it is an integral component of the awareness of those who are on the wrong side of inequality, even if it is usually ignored, hidden, or contested by others."

Bibliography

Abend, Gabriel. "What Are Neural Correlates Neural Correlates Of?" *BioSocieties*, August 11, 2016, 1–24.

Adams, Tim. "How to Spot a Murderer's Brain." *The Guardian*, May 11, 2013, Observer ed., Science section. http://www.theguardian.com/science/2013/may/12/how-to-spot-a-murderers-brain.

Adams, Vincanne, Michelle Murphy, and Adele Clarke. "Anticipation: Technoscience, Life, Affect, Temporality" *Subjectivity* 28 (2009): 246–65.

Adolphs, Ralph. "The Social Brain: Neural Basis of Social Knowledge." *Annual Review of Psychology* 60 (2009): 693–716.

Aguirre, Geoffrey. "Functional Imaging in Behavioral Neurology and Cognitive Neuropsychology." In *Behavioral Neurology and Cognitive Neuropsychology*, edited by Todd Feinberg and Martha Farah, 2nd ed., 85–96. New York: McGraw-Hill, 2003.

———. "Functional Neuroimaging: Technical, Logical, and Social Perspectives." *Hastings Center Report. Interpreting Neuroimages: An Introduction to the Technology and Its Limits* 4, no. 2 (2014): S8–18.

Aharoni, Eyal, Gina M. Vincent, Carla L. Harenski, Vince D. Calhoun, Walter Sinnott-Armstrong, Michael S. Gazzaniga, and Kent A. Kiehl. "Neuroprediction of Future Rearrest." *Proceedings of the National Academy of Sciences of the United States of America* 110, no. 15 (2013): 6223–28.

Alač, Morana. "Digital Scientific Visuals as Fields for Interaction." In *Representation in Scientific Practice Revisited*, edited by Catelijne Coopmans, Janet

Vertesi, Michael E. Lynch, and Steve Woolgar, 61–88. Cambridge, MA: MIT Press, 2014.

———. "Working with Brain Scans: Digital Images and Gestural Interaction in fMRI Laboratory." *Social Studies of Science* 38, no. 4 (2008): 483–508.

Alexander, Michelle. *The New Jim Crow: Mass Incarceration in the Age of Colorblindness.* New York: New Press, 2012.

Allen, Garland. "Old Wine in New Bottles: From Eugenics to Population Control in the Work of Raymond Pearl." In *The Expansion of American Biology,* edited by Ronald Rainger, Keith R. Benson, and Jane Maienschein, 231–61. New Brunswick, NJ: Rutgers University Press, 1991.

American Psychiatric Association. *Diagnostic and Statistical Manual of Mental Disorders.* 4th ed., text rev. Washington, DC: American Psychiatric Association, 2000.

Anderson, Christopher. "NIH, under Fire, Freezes Grant for Conference on Genetics and Crime." *Nature* 358, no. 6385 (1992): 357.

Anderson, Elijah. *Code of the Street: Decency, Violence, and the Moral Life of the Inner City.* Reprint ed. New York: Norton, 2000.

Anderson, Nathaniel E., and Kent A. Kiehl. "The Psychopath Magnetized: Insights from Brain Imaging." *Trends in Cognitive Sciences,* Special Issue: Cognition in Neuropsychiatric Disorders 16, no. 1 (2012): 52–60.

Armenta, Amada. "Racializing Crimmigration: Structural Racism, Colorblindness, and the Institutional Production of Immigrant Criminality" *Sociology of Race and Ethnicity* 3, no. 1 (2017): 82–95.

Arribas-Ayllon, Michael, Srikant Sarangi, and Angus Clarke. "The Micropolitics of Responsibility vis-à-vis Autonomy: Parental Accounts of Childhood Genetic Testing and (Non)Disclosure." *Sociology of Health & Illness* 30, no. 2 (2008): 255–71.

Baldwin, James. "The Negro and the American Promise. Interview by Kenneth Clark." Video, 1963. https://www.pbs.org/video/american-experience-james-baldwin-from-the-negro-and-the-american-promise/.

Balibar, Etienne. "Is There a 'Neo-Racism'?" In *Race, Nation, Class: Ambiguous Identities,* edited by Etienne Balibar and Immanuel Wallerstein, 17–28. London and New York: Verso, 1991.

Barkan, Elazar. *The Retreat of Scientific Racism: Changing Concepts of Race in Britain and the United States between the World Wars.* New York: Cambridge University Press, 1993.

Baron-Cohen, Simon. *The Science of Evil: On Empathy and the Origins of Cruelty.* New York: Basic Books, 2011.

Barrett, Lisa Feldman, Batja Mesquita, Kevin N. Ochsner, and James J. Gross.

"The Experience of Emotion." *Annual Review of Psychology* 58, no. 1 (2006): 373–403.Bartholomew, Allen A., and G. Sutherland. "A Defence of Insanity and the Extra Y Chromosome: R v Hannell." *Australian & New Zealand Journal of Criminology* 2, no. 1 (1969): 29–37.

Bassarath, Lindley. "Neuroimaging Studies of Antisocial Behaviour." *Canadian Journal of Psychiatry* 46, no. 8 (2001): 728–32.

Beaulieu, Anne. "Images Are Not the (Only) Truth: Brain Mapping, Visual Knowledge, and Iconoclasm." *Science, Technology & Human Values* 27, no. 1 (2002): 53–86.

Beaver, Kevin M. *Biosocial Criminology: A Primer.* 3rd ed. Dubuque, IA: Kendall Hunt Publishing, 2016.

Becker, Peter. "The Criminologists' Gaze at the Underworld." In *Criminals and Their Scientists: The History of Criminology in International Perspective,* edited by Peter Becker and Richard F. Wetzell, 105–33. 1st ed. Cambridge, UK and New York: Cambridge University Press, 2006.

———. "New Monsters on the Block?: On the Return of Biological Explanations of Crime and Violence." In *Cuerpos Anómalos,* edited by Max S. Hering Torres, 265–99. Bogotá: Universidad Nacional de Colombia, 2008.

Becker, Peter, and Richard F. Wetzell, eds. *Criminals and Their Scientists: The History of Criminology in International Perspective.* 1st ed. Cambridge, UK and New York: Cambridge University Press, 2006.

Beckwith, Jonathan. "The Persistent Influence of Failed Scientific Ideas." In *Genetic Explanations: Sense and Nonsense,* edited by Sheldon Krimsky and Jeremy Gruber, 173–85. Cambridge, MA: Harvard University Press, 2013.

Benjamin, Ruha. "Innovating Inequity: If Race Is a Technology, Postracialism Is the Genius Bar." *Ethnic and Racial Studies* 39, no. 13 (2016): 2227–34.

Berkman, Elliot T., and Emily B. Falk. "Beyond Brain Mapping: Using Neural Measures to Predict Real-World Outcomes." *Current Directions in Psychological Science* 22, no. 1 (2013): 45–50.

Berkowitz, Leonard. *Aggression: Its Causes, Consequences, and Control.* New York: McGraw-Hill, 1993.

Berman, Elizabeth Popp. *Creating the Market University: How Academic Science Became an Economic Engine.* Princeton, NJ: Princeton University Press, 2011.

Blair, James R. "Neuroimaging of Psychopathy and Antisocial Behavior: A Targeted Review." *Current Psychiatry Reports* 12, no. 1 (2010): 76–82.

———. "Psychopathy: Cognitive and Neural Dysfunction." *Dialogues in Clinical Neuroscience* 15, no. 2 (2013): 181–90.

———. "Too Much of a Good Thing: Increased Grey Matter in Boys with Conduct Problems and Callous-Unemotional Traits." *Brain* 132, no. 4 (2009): 831–32.

Blais, Julie, Adelle E. Forth, and Robert D. Hare. "Examining the Interrater Reliability of the Hare Psychopathy Checklist—Revised across a Large Sample of Trained Raters." *Psychological Assessment* 29, no. 6 (2017): 762–75.

2Blake, Pamela, and Jordan Grafman. "The Neurobiology of Aggression." *Lancet (London, England)* 364 Suppl. 1 (2004): s12–13.

Blakemore, Sarah-Jayne. "The Social Brain in Adolescence." *Nature Reviews Neuroscience* 9, no. 4 (2008): 267–77.

Bliss, Catherine. *Race Decoded: The Genomic Fight for Social Justice.* Stanford, CA: Stanford University Press, 2012.

———. *Social by Nature: The Promise and Peril of Sociogenomics.* Stanford, CA: Stanford University Press, 2018.

Bloch, Michael H., and Ahmad Qawasmi. "Omega-3 Fatty Acid Supplementation for the Treatment of Children with Attention-Deficit/Hyperactivity Disorder Symptomatology: Systematic Review and Meta-Analysis." *Journal of the American Academy of Child and Adolescent Psychiatry* 50, no. 10 (2011): 991–1000.

Blumer, Herbert. *Symbolic Interactionism: Perspective and Method.* Berkeley: University of California Press, 1986.

Bobo, Lawrence, James R. Kluegel, and Ryan A. Smith. "Laissez-Faire Racism: The Crystallization of a 'Kindler, Genter' Anti-Black Ideology." In *Racial Attitudes in the 1990s: Continuity and Change,* edited by Jack Martin and Steven A. Tuch, 15–42. Westport, CT: Praeger, 1997.

Boffey, Philip M., Luther J. Carter, and Andrew Hamilton. "Nixon Budget: Science Funding Remains Tight." *Science* 167, no. 3919 (1970): 845–48.

Bonilla-Silva, Eduardo. *Racism without Racists: Color-Blind Racism and the Persistence of Racial Inequality in America.* 2nd ed.. Lanham, MD: Rowman & Littlefield Publishers, 2006.

———. "Rethinking Racism: Toward a Structural Interpretation." *American Sociological Review* 62, no. 3 (1997): 465–80.

Bourdieu, Pierre. "The Specificity of the Scientific Field and the Social Conditions of the Progress of Reason." *Social Science Information* 14, no. 6 (1975): 19–47.

Bowker, Geoffrey C., and Susan L. Star. *Sorting Things Out: Classification and Its Consequences.* Cambridge, MA: MIT Press, 1999.

Broer, Tineke, and Martyn Pickersgill. "Targeting Brains, Producing Responsibilities: The Use of Neuroscience within British Social Policy." *Social Science & Medicine* 132 (2015): 54–61.

Brown, Michael K., Martin Carnoy, Elliott Currie, Troy Duster, and David B. Oppenheimer. *Whitewashing Race: The Myth of a Color-Blind Society.* Berkeley: University of California Press, 2003.

Brown, Simone. *Dark Matters: On the Surveillance of Blackness*. Durham, NC: Duke University Press, 2015.

Brunner, Han G. "Monoamine Oxidase and Behaviour." *Annals of Medicine* 27, no. 4 (1995): 431–32.

Brunner, Han G., M. Nelen, X. O. Breakefield, H. H. Ropers, and B. A. van Oost. "Abnormal Behavior Associated with a Point Mutation in the Structural Gene for Monoamine Oxidase A." *Science* 262, no. 5133 (1993): 578–80.

Buchsbaum, M. S., K. H. Nuechterlein, R. J. Haier, J. Wu, N. Sicotte, E. Hazlett, R. Asarnow, S. Potkin, and S. Guich. "Glucose Metabolic Rate in Normals and Schizophrenics during the Continuous Performance Test Assessed by Positron Emission Tomography." *British Journal of Psychiatry: The Journal of Mental Science* 156 (1990): 216–27.

Buckholtz, Joshua W., and Andreas Meyer-Lindenberg. "Gene-Brain Associations: The Example of MAOA." In *The Neurobiological Basis of Violence: Science and Rehabilitation*, edited by Sheilagh Hodgins, Essi Viding, and Anna Plodowski, 265–85. Oxford: Oxford University Press, 2009.

———. "MAOA and the Bioprediction of Antisocial Behavior: Science Fact and Science Fiction." In *Bioprediction, Biomarkers, and Bad Behavior: Scientific, Legal, and Ethical Challenges*, edited by Ilina Singh, Walter P. Sinnott-Armstrong, and Julian Savulecu, 131–52. New York: Oxford University Press, 2014.

Bufkin, Jana L., and Vickie R. Luttrell. "Neuroimaging Studies of Aggressive and Violent Behavior: Current Findings and Implications for Criminology and Criminal Justice." *Trauma, Violence & Abuse* 6, no. 2 (2005): 176–91.

Burke, Meghan. *Colorblind Racism*. 1st ed. Medford, MA: Polity, 2019.

Burt, Callie H., and Ronald L. Simons. "Pulling Back the Curtain on Heritability Studies: Biosocial Criminology in the Postgenomic Era." *Criminology* 52, no. 2 (2014): 223–62.

Bush, George H. W. "Decade of the Brain: Presidential Proclamation 6158." Presidential Proclamation presented at the Project on the Decade of the Brain, The White House, July 17, 1990. https://www.loc.gov/loc/brain/proclaim.html.

Byrd, Amy L., and Stephen B. Manuck. "MAOA, Childhood Maltreatment, and Antisocial Behavior: Meta-Analysis of a Gene-Environment Interaction." *Biological Psychiatry* 75, no. 1 (2014): 9–17.

Canguilhem, Georges. *The Normal and the Pathological*. Translated by Carolyn R. Fawcett. New York: Zone Books, 1991.

Caplan, Lincoln. *The Insanity Defense and the Trial of John W Hinckley, Jr.* Boston: David R. Godine, 1984.

Carey, Gregory, and Irving I. Gottesman. "Genetics and Antisocial Behavior:

Substance versus Sound Bytes." *Politics and the Life Sciences: The Journal of the Association for Politics and the Life Sciences* 15, no. 1 (1996): 88–90.

Carrier, Nicolas, and Kevin Walby. "Ptolemizing Lombroso: The Pseudo-Revolution of Biosocial Criminology." *Journal of Theoretical and Philosophical Criminology* 6, no. 1 (2014): 1–45.

Cases, O., I. Seif, J. Grimsby, P. Gaspar, K. Chen, S. Pournin, U. Müller, M. Aguet, C. Babinet, and J. C. Shih. "Aggressive Behavior and Altered Amounts of Brain Serotonin and Norepinephrine in Mice Lacking MAOA." *Science* 268, no. 5218 (1995): 1763–66.

Caspi, Avshalom, Joseph McClay, Terrie E. Moffitt, Jonathan Mill, Judy Martin, Ian W. Craig, Alan Taylor, and Richie Poulton. "Role of Genotype in the Cycle of Violence in Maltreated Children." *Science* 297, no. 5582 (2002): 851–54.

Castel, Robert. "From Dangerousness to Risk." In *The Foucault Effect: Studies in Governmentality : With Two Lectures by and an Interview with Michel Foucault*, edited by Graham Burchell, Colin Gordon, and Peter M. Miller, 281–98. Chicago: University of Chicago Press, 1991.

Chorover, Stephen. "Violence: A Localizable Problem?" In *Biology, Crime and Ethics: A Study of Biological Explanations for Criminal Behavior*, edited by Frank H. Marsh and Janet Katz, 255–70. Cincinnati: Anderson, 1984.

Clarke, Adele E., and Monica J. Casper. "From Simple Technology to Complex Arena: Classification of Pap Smears, 1917–90." *Medical Anthropology Quarterly* 10, no. 4 (1996): 601–23.

Clarke, Adele E., and Joan H. Fujimura. *The Right Tools for the Job: At Work in Twentieth-Century Life Sciences*. Princeton, NJ: Princeton University Press, 1992.

Clarke, Adele E., Laura Mamo, Jennifer Ruth Fosket, Jennifer R. Fishman, and Janet K. Shim, eds. *Biomedicalization: Technoscience, Health, and Illness in the U.S.* Durham, NC: Duke University Press, 2010.

Clarke, Adele E., Janet K. Shim, Laura Mamo, Jennifer Ruth Fosket, and Jennifer R. Fishman. "Biomedicalization: Technoscientific Transformations of Health, Illness, and U.S. Biomedicine." *American Sociological Review* 68, no. 2 (2003): 161–94.

Coccaro, Emil F. "Intermittent Explosive Disorder: Development of Integrated Research Criteria for Diagnostic and Statistical Manual of Mental Disorders, Fifth Edition." *Comprehensive Psychiatry* 52, no. 2 (2011): 119–25.

Coccaro, Emil F., Michael S. McCloskey, Daniel A. Fitzgerald, and K. Luan Phan. "Amygdala and Orbitofrontal Reactivity to Social Threat in Individuals with Impulsive Aggression." *Biological Psychiatry* 62, no. 2 (2007): 168–78.

Coleman, Lee S. "Perspectives on the Medical Research of Violence." *American Journal of Orthopsychiatry* 44, no. 5 (1974): 675–87.

Conley, Dalton, and Jason Fletcher. *The Genome Factor: What the Social Ge-nomics Revolution Reveals about Ourselves, Our History, and the Future.* Princeton, NJ: Princeton University Press, 2017.

Connell, R. W. *Masculinities.* Berkeley: University of California Press, 2005.

Connell, R. W., and James W. Messerschmidt. "Hegemonic Masculinity: Re-thinking the Concept." *Gender and Society* 19, no. 6 (2005): 829–59.

Conrad, Peter, and Joseph W. Schneider. *Deviance and Medicalization: From Badness to Sickness.* Philadelphia: Temple University Press, 1992.

Cornel, Tabea. "Something Old, Something New, Something Pseudo, Some-thing True: Pejorative and Deferential References to Phrenology since 1840." *Proceedings of the American Philosophical Society* 161, no. 4 (2017): 299–332.

Craig, Ian W. "The Role of Monoamine Oxidase A, MAOA, in the Aetiology of An-tisocial Behaviour: The Importance of Gene-Environment Interactions." *Novartis Foundation Symposium* 268 (2005): 227–37; discussion 237–41, 242–53.

Damasio, Antonio. *Descartes' Error: Emotion, Reason, and the Human Brain.* New York: Penguin, 2005.

Damasio, H., T. Grabowski, R. Frank, A. M. Galaburda, and A. R. Damasio. "The Return of Phineas Gage: Clues about the Brain from the Skull of a Famous Patient." *Science* 264, no. 5162 (1994): 1102–5.

Dana Foundation. "A Decade after the Decade of the Brain: Compilation." New York: Dana Foundation, 2010.

Davidson, Richard J., Katherine M. Putnam, and Christine L. Larson. "Dysfunc-tion in the Neural Circuitry of Emotion Regulation—A Possible Prelude to Violence." *Science* 289, no. 5479 (2000): 591–94.

De Vos, Jan. "What Is Critique in the Era of the Neurosciences?" In *Neuroscience and Critique: Exploring the Limits of the Neurological Turn,* edited by Jan De Vos and Ed Pluth, 22–40. New York: Routledge, 2016.

Decety, Jean, Kalina J. Michalska, Yuko Akitsuki, and Benjamin B. Lahey. "Atyp-ical Empathic Responses in Adolescents with Aggressive Conduct Disorder: A Functional MRI Investigation." *Biological Psychology* 80, no. 2 (2009): 203.

Dick, Philip K. *Selected Stories of Philip K. Dick.* 1st ed. Boston: Houghton Mifflin Harcourt, 2013.

Diener, Ed. "Neuroimaging: Voodoo, New Phrenology, or Scientific Break-through? Introduction to Special Section on fMRI." *Perspectives on Psycho-logical Science* 5, no. 6 (2010): 714–15.

DiLalla, Lisabeth F., and Irving I. Gottesman. "Biological and Genetic Contrib-utors to Violence: Widom's Untold Tale." *Psychological Bulletin* 109, no. 1 (1991): 125–29.

Dolan, R. J. "Neuroimaging of Cognition." *Neuron* 60, no. 3 (2008): 496–502.

Donaldson, David I. "Parsing Brain Activity with fMRI and Mixed Designs: What Kind of a State Is Neuroimaging In?" *Trends in Neurosciences* 27, no. 8 (2004): 442–44.

Du Bois, W.E.B. *The Souls of Black Folk: Essays and Sketches.* 1903. Reprint, New York: Vintage, 1990.

Dumit, Joseph. "The Fragile Unity of Neuroscience." In *Neuroscience and Critique: Exploring the Limits of the Neurological Turn*, edited by Jan De Vos and Ed Pluth, 223–30. New York: Routledge, 2016.

———. "How (Not) to Do Things with Brain Images." In *Representation in Scientific Practice Revisited*, edited by Catelijne Coopmans, Janet Vertesi, Michael E. Lynch, and Steve Woolgar, 291–313. Cambridge, MA: MIT Press, 2014.

———. *Picturing Personhood: Brain Scans and Biomedical Identity.* Princeton, NJ: Princeton University Press, 2004.

Dupras, Charles, and Vardit Ravitsky. "Epigenetics in the Neoliberal 'Regime of Truth': A Biopolitical Perspective on Knowledge Translation." *Hastings Center Report* 46, no. 1 (2016): 26–35.

Durkheim, Emile. *The Division of Labor in Society.* Translated by Lewis A. Coser. New York: Simon and Schuster, 1895.

Duster, Troy. *Backdoor to Eugenics.* 2nd ed. New York: Routledge, 2003.

———. "Behavioral Genetics and the Link between Crime, Violence, and Race," edited by Erik Parens, Audrey R. Chapman, and Nancy Press, 150–75. Baltimore: John Hopkins University Press, 2006.

———. "Comparative Perspectives and Competing Explanations: Taking on the Newly Configured Reductionist Challenge to Sociology." *American Sociological Review* 71, no. 1 (2006): 1–15.

———. "Explaining Differential Trust of DNA Forensic Technology: Grounded Assessment or Inexplicable Paranoia?" *Journal of Law, Medicine & Ethics* 34, no. 2 (2006): 293–300.

———. "Lessons from History: Why Race and Ethnicity Have Played a Major Role in Biomedical Research." *Journal of Law, Medicine & Ethics* 34, no. 3 (2006): 487–96.

"Ebony Magazine, Letters to the Editor—Brain Surgery." *Ebony*, May 1973.

"Ebony Magazine, Letters to the Editor—Psychosurgery." *Ebony*, November 1973.

Epstein, Steven. *Inclusion: The Politics of Difference in Medical Research.* Chicago: University of Chicago Press, 2009.

———. "The Rise of 'Recruitmentology': Clinical Research, Racial Knowledge, and the Politics of Inclusion and Difference." *Social Studies of Science* 38, no. 5 (2008): 801–32.

Erlich, Yaniv, Tal Shor, Itsik Pe'er, and Shai Carmi. "Identity Inference of Genomic

Data Using Long-Range Familial Searches." *Science* 362, no. 6415 (2018): 690–94.

Ervin, Frank. "Violence and Brain Disease." *Journal of the American Medical Association (JAMA)* 226, no. 12 (1973): 1463–64.

Etchegary, Holly, Fiona Miller, Sonya deLaat, Brenda Wilson, June Carroll, and Mario Cappelli. "Decision-Making about Inherited Cancer Risk: Exploring Dimensions of Genetic Responsibility." *Journal of Genetic Counseling* 18, no. 3 (2009): 252–64.

Eubanks, Virginia. *Automating Inequality: How High-Tech Tools Profile, Police, and Punish the Poor.* New York: St. Martin's, 2018.

Eysenck, Hans Jürgen. *Crime and Personality.* Routledge & K. Paul, 1977.

———. *Race, Intelligence, and Education.* London: Maurice Temple Smith, 1971.

Faigman, David, John Monahan, and Christopher Slobogin. "Group to Individual (G2i) Inference in Scientific Expert Testimony." *University of Chicago Law Review* 81, no. 2 (2014): 417–80.

Falk, Emily B., Elliot T. Berkman, and Matthew D. Lieberman. "From Neural Responses to Population Behavior: Neural Focus Group Predicts Population-Level Media Effects." *Psychological Science* 23, no. 5 (2012): 439–45.

Farahany, Nita A. "Neuroscience and Behavioral Genetics in US Criminal Law: An Empirical Analysis." *Journal of Law and the Biosciences* 2, no. 3 (2015): 485–509.

Fassin, Didier. *Life: A Critical User's Manual.* 1st ed. Cambridge, UK: Polity, 2018.

Feagin, Joe R. *Systemic Racism: A Theory of Oppression.* New York: Routledge, 2006.

Ficks, Courtney A., and Irwin D. Waldman. "Candidate Genes for Aggression and Antisocial Behavior: A Meta-Analysis of Association Studies of the 5HTTLPR and MAOA-uVNTR." *Behavior Genetics* 44, no. 5 (2014): 427–44.

Fink, Arthur E. *Causes of Crime: Biological Theories in the United States, 1800–1915.* Philadelphia: University of Pennsylvania Press, 1938.

Fishbein, Diana. *Biobehavioral Perspectives on Criminology.* 1st ed. Australia; Belmont, CA: Wadsworth Publishing, 2000.

Fleck, Ludwik. *Genesis and Development of a Scientific Fact.* Edited by Thaddeus J. Trenn and Robert K. Merton. Translated by Frederick Bradley. Chicago: University of Chicago Press, 1981.

Foucault, Michel. *The Birth of the Clinic: An Archaeology of Medical Perception.* New York: Vintage, 1994.

———. *Discipline and Punish: The Birth of the Prison.* New York: Vintage, 1995.

———. *Security, Territory, Population: Lectures at the College De France, 1977-78.* New York: Palgrave Macmillan, 2007.

Frick, Paul J., and Essi Viding. "Antisocial Behavior from a Developmental Psychopathology Perspective." *Development and Psychopathology* 21, no. 4 (2009): 1111–31.

Friston, Karl. "Beyond Phrenology: What Can Neuroimaging Tell Us about Distributed Circuitry?" *Annual Review of Neuroscience* 25, no. 1 (2002): 221–50.

Frith, Chris D. "The Social Brain?" *Philosophical Transactions of the Royal Society B: Biological Sciences* 362, no. 1480 (2007): 671–78.

Fujimura, Joan H. "Future Imaginaries: Genome Scientists as Sociocultural Entrepreneurs." In *Genetic Nature/Culture: Anthropology and Science beyond the Two-Culture Divide*, edited by Alan H. Goodman, Deborah Heath, and M. Susan Lindee, 176–99. Berkeley: University of California Press, 2003.

Fujimura, Joan H., Troy Duster, and Ramya Rajagopalan. "Introduction: Race, Genetics, and Disease: Questions of Evidence, Matters of Consequence." *Social Studies of Science* 38, no. 5 (2008): 643–56.

Fullwiley, Duana. "The Molecularization of Race: Institutionalizing Human Difference in Pharmacogenetics Practice." *Science as Culture* 16, no. 1 (2007): 1–30.

Gabbidon, Shaun L., ed. *Criminological Perspectives on Race and Crime*. New York: Routledge, 2015.

Gard, Arianna M., Rebecca Waller, Daniel S. Shaw, Erika E. Forbes, Ahmad R. Hariri, and Luke W. Hyde. "The Long Reach of Early Adversity: Parenting, Stress, and Neural Pathways to Antisocial Behavior in Adulthood." *Biological Psychiatry: Cognitive Neuroscience and Neuroimaging* 2, no. 7 (2017): 582–90.

Gazzaniga, Michael S. "What Is Cognitive Neuroscience?" In *A Judge's Guide to Neuroscience: A Concise Introduction*, 2–4. Santa Barbara, CA: SAGE Center for the Study of the Mind, 2010.

Gibbons, Ann. "Tracking the Evolutionary History of a 'Warrior' Gene." *Science* 304, no. 5672 (2004): 818.

Gillett, Grant, and Armon J. Tamatea. "The Warrior Gene: Epigenetic Considerations." *New Genetics and Society* 31, no. 1 (2012): 41–53.

Gilroy, Paul. *There Ain't No Black in the Union Jack*. 2nd ed. London: Routledge, 2002.

Gläser, Jochen, and Grit Laudel. "Governing Science: How Science Policy Shapes Research Content." *European Journal of Sociology / Archives Européennes de Sociologie* 57, no. 1 (2016): 117–68.

Glenn, Andrea L., and Adrian Raine. "Neurocriminology: Implications for the Punishment, Prediction, and Prevention of Criminal Behaviour." *Nature Reviews. Neuroscience* 15, no. 1 (2014): 54–63.

———. *Psychopathy: An Introduction to Biological Findings and Their Implications.* New York: NYU Press, 2014.

Goldberg, David Theo. *The Racial State.* 1st ed. Malden, MA: Wiley-Blackwell, 2001.

———. *The Threat of Race: Reflections on Racial Neoliberalism.* 1st ed. Malden, MA: Wiley-Blackwell, 2008.

Goldman, David, and Alexandra A. Rosser. "MAOA-Environment Interactions: Results May Vary." *Biological Psychiatry* 75, no. 1 (2014): 2–3.

Goosby, Bridget J., Jacob E. Cheadle, and Colter Mitchell. "Stress-Related Bio-social Mechanisms of Discrimination and African American Health Inequities." *Annual Review of Sociology* 44, no. 1 (2018): 319–40.

Gould, Stephen Jay. *The Mismeasure of Man.* New York: Norton, 2006.

Greely, Henry T., and Nita A. Farahany. "Neuroscience and the Criminal Justice System." *Annual Review of Criminology* 2, no. 1 (2019): 451–71.

Greely, Henry T., Daniel P. Riordan, Nanibaa' A. Garrison, and Joanna L. Mountain. "Family Ties: The Use of DNA Offender Databases to Catch Offenders' Kin." *Journal of Law, Medicine & Ethics* 34, no. 2 (2006): 248–62.

Gunderman, Richard B. *X-Ray Vision: The Evolution of Medical Imaging and Its Human Significance.* New York: Oxford University Press, 2013.

Haberstick, Brett C., Jeffrey M. Lessem, Christian J. Hopfer, Andrew Smolen, Marissa A. Ehringer, David Timberlake, and John K. Hewitt. "Monoamine Oxidase A (MAOA) and Antisocial Behaviors in the Presence of Childhood and Adolescent Maltreatment." *American Journal of Medical Genetics. Part B, Neuropsychiatric Genetics: The Official Publication of the International Society of Psychiatric Genetics* 135B, no. 1 (2005): 59–64.

Hackett, Edward J. "Funding and Academic Research in the Life Sciences: Results of an Exploratory Study." *Science & Technology Studies* 5, no. 3/4 (1987): 134–47.

Hacking, Ian. "Degeneracy, Criminal Behavior, and Looping." In *Genetics and Criminal Behavior,* edited by David Wasserman and Robert Wachbroit, 141–68. Cambridge, UK: Cambridge University Press, 2001.

———. *The Social Construction of What?* Cambridge, MA: Harvard University Press, 1999.

Hall, Stuart. "Who Needs Identity?" In *Identity: A Reader,* edited by Paul du Gay, Jessica Evans, and Peter Redman, 15–30. 1st ed. London; Thousand Oaks, CA: SAGE, 2000.

Halpern, Sue. "The Neuroscience of Picking a Presidential Candidate." *The New Yorker,* February 3, 2020. https://www.newyorker.com/tech/annals-of-technology/the-neuroscience-of-picking-a-presidential-candidate.

Hamid, Nafees. "What I Learned from Scanning the Brains of Potential Terrorists." *New York Times,* March 2, 2020, Opinion section. https://www.nytimes.com/2020/03/02/opinion/domestic-terrorism-jihadists.html.

Hamid, Nafees, Clara Pretus, Scott Atran, Molly J. Crockett, Jeremy Ginges, Hammad Sheikh, Adolf Tobeña et al. "Neuroimaging 'Will to Fight' for Sacred Values: An Empirical Case Study with Supporters of an Al Qaeda Associate." *Royal Society Open Science* 6, no. 6 (2019): 1–13.

Harcourt, Bernard E. "Risk as a Proxy for Race: The Dangers of Risk Assessment." *Federal Sentencing Reporter* 27, no. 4 (2015): 237–43.

Hare, Robert D. "The Hare PCL-R: Some Issues Concerning Its Use and Misuse." *Legal and Criminological Psychology* 3 (1998): 99–119.

Harlow, John M. "Recovery from the Passage of an Iron Bar through the Head (Originally Published 1868)." *History of Psychiatry* 4, no. 14 (1993): 274–81.

Hatch, Anthony Ryan. *Blood Sugar: Racial Pharmacology and Food Justice in Black America.* 1st ed. Minneapolis: University of Minnesota Press, 2016.

Hawkins, Darnell F., ed. *Ethnicity, Race, and Crime: Perspectives across Time and Place.* Albany: State University of New York Press, 1995.

Haynes, John-Dylan, and Geraint Rees. "Decoding Mental States from Brain Activity in Humans." *Nature Reviews Neuroscience* 7, no. 7 (2006): 523–34.

Heinemann, Torsten, Thomas Lemke, and Barbara Prainsack. "Risky Profiles: Societal Dimensions of Forensic Uses of DNA Profiling Technologies." *New Genetics and Society* 31, no. 3 (2012): 249–58.

Herbert, Wray. "Politics of Biology: How the Nature vs. Nurture Debate Shapes Public Policy and Our View of Ourselves." *U.S. News & World Report* 122, no. 15 (1997): 72–79.

Heron, Melonie. "Deaths: Leading Causes for 2017." National Vital Statistics Reports. Hyattsville, MD: National Center for Health Statistics, 2019.

Herpertz, Sabine C., Thomas Huebner, Ivo Marx, Timo D. Vloet, Gereon R. Fink, Tony Stoecker, N. Jon Shah, Kerstin Konrad, and Beate Herpertz-Dahlmann. "Emotional Processing in Male Adolescents with Childhood-Onset Conduct Disorder." *Journal of Child Psychology and Psychiatry, and Allied Disciplines* 49, no. 7 (2008): 781–91.

Holmes, Avram J., and Lauren M. Patrick. "The Myth of Optimality in Clinical Neuroscience." *Trends in Cognitive Sciences* 22, no. 3 (2018): 241–57.

Horn, David G. "Making Criminologists: Tools, Techniques, and the Production of Scientific Authority." In *Criminals and Their Scientists: The History of Criminology in International Perspective*, edited by Peter Becker and Richard F. Wetzell, 317–36. 1st ed. Cambridge, UK: Cambridge University Press, 2006.

Hyde, Luke W., Daniel S. Shaw, Laura Murray, Arianna Gard, Ahmad R. Hariri, and Erika E. Forbes. "Dissecting the Role of Amygdala Reactivity in Antisocial Behavior in a Sample of Young, Low-Income, Urban Men." *Clinical*

Psychological Science: A Journal of the Association for Psychological Science 4, no. 3 (2016): 527–44.

Jacobs, P. A., M. Brunton, M. M. Melville, R. P. Brittain, and W. F. McClemont. "Aggressive Behavior, Mental Sub-Normality and the XYY Male." *Nature* 208, no. 5017 (1965): 1351–52.

James, Joy. *Resisting State Violence: Radicalicism, Gender, and Race in U.S. Culture*. Minneapolis, MN: University of Minnesota Press, 1996.

Jasanoff, Sheila. "The Idiom of Co-Production." In *States of Knowledge: The Co-Production of Science and the Social Order*, edited by Sheila Jasanoff, 1–12. New York: Routledge, 2004.

Jasanoff, Sheila, and Sang-Hyun Kim. "Containing the Atom: Sociotechnical Imaginaries and Nuclear Power in the United States and South Korea." *Minerva* 47, no. 2 (2009): 119–46.

Jeffery, C. R. "Criminology as an Interdisciplinary Behavioral Science." *Criminology* 16, no. 2 (1978): 149–69.

Jones, Owen D., and Francis X. Shen. "Law and Neuroscience in the United States." In *International Neurolaw: A Comparative Analysis*, edited by Tade Matthias Spranger, 349–80. Berlin, Heidelberg: Springer Berlin Heidelberg, 2012.

Jordan-Young, Rebecca M., and Katrina Karkazis. *Testosterone: An Unauthorized Biography*. 1st ed. Cambridge, MA: Harvard University Press, 2019.

Joyce, Kelly A. *Magnetic Appeal: MRI and the Myth of Transparency*. Ithaca, NY: Cornell University Press, 2008.

———. "Neuroimaging Production in Clinical Practice." In *Sociological Reflections on the Neurosciences*, edited by Martyn Pickersgill and Ira Van Keulen, 13:75–98. Advances in Medical Sociology. 1st ed. Bingley: Emerald Group Publishing, 2011.

Kahn, Jonathan. *Race on the Brain: What Implicit Bias Gets Wrong about the Struggle for Racial Justice*. New York: Columbia University Press, 2018.

Karkazis, Katrina and Rebecca Jordan-Young. 2020. "Sensing Race as a Ghost Variable in Science, Technology, and Medicine." *Science, Technology, & Human Values*. 45 (5):763–78.

Kevles, Bettyann. *Naked to the Bone: Medical Imaging in the Twentieth Century*. New York: Basic Books, 1998.

Kiehl, Kent A. *The Psychopath Whisperer: The Science of Those without Conscience*. New York: Broadway Books, 2014.

Kiehl, Kent A., Nathaniel E. Anderson, Eyal Aharoni, J. Michael Maurer, Keith A. Harenski, Vikram Rao, Eric D. Claus et al. "Age of Gray Matters: Neuroprediction of Recidivism." *NeuroImage: Clinical* 19 (2018): 813–23.

Kiernan, Laura A. "Hinckley Judge Reverses Himself, Admits Pictures of Defendant's Brain." *Washington Post*, June 2, 1982.

Kirby, A., A. Woodward, S. Jackson, Y. Wang, and M. A. Crawford. "A Double-Blind, Placebo-Controlled Study Investigating the Effects of Omega-3 Supplementation in Children Aged 8–10 Years from a Mainstream School Population." *Research in Developmental Disabilities* 31, no. 3 (2010): 718–30.

Kirkpatrick, Sharon I., Lynn McIntyre, and Melissa L. Potestio. "Child Hunger and Long-Term Adverse Consequences for Health." *Archives of Pediatrics & Adolescent Medicine* 164, no. 8 (2010): 754–62.

Knorr-Cetina, Karin. *Epistemic Cultures: How the Sciences Make Knowledge.* Cambridge, MA: Harvard University Press, 1999.

Koenig, Barbara, Sandra Soo-Jin Lee, and Sarah S. Richardson. *Revisiting Race in a Genomic Age.* New Brunswick, NJ: Rutgers University Press, 2008.

Kosik, Kenneth S. "Beyond Phrenology, at Last." *Nature Reviews Neuroscience* 4, no. 3 (2003): 234–39.

Kubota, Jennifer T., Mahzarin R. Banaji, and Elizabeth A. Phelps. "The Neuroscience of Race." *Nature Neuroscience* 15, no. 7 (2012): 940–48.

Kuhn, Thomas S. *The Structure of Scientific Revolutions.* 3rd ed. Chicago: University of Chicago Press, 1996.

Lakatos, I. "Falsification and the Methodology of Scientific Research Programmes." In *Criticism and the Growth of Knowledge: Proceedings of the International Colloquium in the Philosophy of Science, London, 1965,* edited by Alan Musgrave and Imre Lakatos, 4:91–196. Cambridge: Cambridge University Press, 1970.

Landecker, Hannah. "Food as Exposure: Nutritional Epigenetics and the New Metabolism." *Biosocieties* 6, no. 2 (2011): 167–94.

Landecker, Hannah, and Aaron Panofsky. "From Social Structure to Gene Regulation, and Back: A Critical Introduction to Environmental Epigenetics for Sociology." *Annual Review of Sociology* 39 (2013): 333–57.

Lappé, Martine. "The Maternal Body as Environment in Autism Science." *Social Studies of Science* 46, no. 5 (2016): 675–700.

Larregue, Julien. *Héréditaire: L'éternel retour des théories biologiques du crime.* Paris: Éditions du Seuil, 2020.

Larregue, Julien, and Oliver Rollins. "Biosocial Criminology and the Mismeasure of Race." *Ethnic and Racial Studies* 42, no. 12 (2019): 1990–2007.

Latour, Bruno, and Steve Woolgar. *Laboratory Life: The Construction of Scientific Facts.* Princeton, NJ: Princeton University Press, 1979.

Lea, Rod, and Geoffrey Chambers. "Monoamine Oxidase, Addiction, and the

'Warrior' Gene Hypothesis." *New Zealand Medical Journal* 120, no. 1250 (2007): 5–10.

Lee, Catherine, and Torsten H. Voigt. "DNA Testing for Family Reunification and the Limits of Biological Truth." *Science, Technology, & Human Values,* July 17, 2019, Online First.

Lemke, Thomas. *Biopolitics: An Advanced Introduction.* New York: NYU Press, 2011.

Lewis, Jason E., David DeGusta, Marc R. Meyer, Janet M. Monge, Alan E. Mann, and Ralph L. Holloway. "The Mismeasure of Science: Stephen Jay Gould versus Samuel George Morton on Skulls and Bias." *PLOS Biology* 9, no. 6 (2011): e1001071.

Lewis, LaVonna Blair, David C. Sloane, Lori Miller Nascimento, Allison L. Diamant, Joyce Jones Guinyard, Antronette K. Yancey, and Gwendolyn Flynn. "African Americans' Access to Healthy Food Options in South Los Angeles Restaurants." *American Journal of Public Health* 95, no. 4 (2005): 668–73.

Lieberman, Matthew D. *Social: Why Our Brains Are Wired to Connect.* New York: Crown, 2013.

Lindesmith, Alfred, and Yale Levin. "The Lombrosian Myth in Criminology." *American Journal of Sociology* 42, no. 5 (1937): 653–71.

Loeber, Rolf, and Dustin Pardini. "Neurobiology and the Development of Violence: Common Assumptions and Controversies." *Philosophical Transactions of the Royal Society of London. Series B, Biological Sciences* 363, no. 1503 (2008): 2491–2503.

Lombroso, Cesare. *Criminal Man.* Translated by Mary Gibson and Nicole Hahn Rafter. 1876. Reprint, Durham, NC: Duke University Press, 2006.

Lupton, Deborah. "Foucault and the Medicalisation Critique." In *Foucault, Health, and Medicine,* edited by Robin Bunton and Alan Petersen, 94–110. London: Routledge, 1997.

Ly, Martina, Julian C. Motzkin, Carissa L. Philippi, Gregory R. Kirk, Joseph P. Newman, Kent A. Kiehl, and Michael Koenigs. "Cortical Thinning in Psychopathy." *American Journal of Psychiatry* 169, no. 7 (2012): 743–49.

Lynam, Donald R., and David D. Vachon. "Antisocial Personality Disorder in DSM-5: Missteps and Missed Opportunities." *Personality Disorders: Theory, Research, and Treatment* 3, no. 4 (2012): 483–95.

Lynch, Michael E. "Representation in Formation." In *Representation in Scientific Practice Revisited,* edited by Catelijne Coopmans, Janet Vertesi, Michael E. Lynch, and Steve Woolgar, 323–27. Cambridge, MA: MIT Press, 2014.

Malterer, Melanie B., Scott O. Lilienfeld, Craig S. Neumann, and Joseph P.

Newman. "Concurrent Validity of the Psychopathic Personality Inventory with Offender and Community Samples." *Assessment* 17, no. 1 (2010): 3–15.

Mansfield, Becky, and Julie Guthman. "Epigenetic Life: Biological Plasticity, Abnormality, and New Configurations of Race and Reproduction." *Cultural Geographies* 22, no. 1 (2015): 3–20.

Marcus, George E. *Technoscientific Imaginaries: Conversations, Profiles, and Memoirs.* Chicago: University of Chicago Press, 1995.

Mark, Vernon H. "Social and Ethical Issues: Brain Surgery in Aggressive Epileptics." *Hastings Center Report* 3, no. 1 (1973): 1–5.

Mark, Vernon H., William H. Sweet, and Frank R. Ervin. "Role of Brain Disease in Riots and Urban Violence." *Journal of the American Medical Association (JAMA)* 201, no. 11 (1967): 895.

———. "Role of Brain Disease in Riots and Urban Violence." *Journal of the American Medical Association (JAMA)* 203, no. 5 (1968): 368–69.

Marsh, Abigail. *The Fear Factor: How One Emotion Connects Altruists, Psychopaths, and Everyone In-Between.* 1st ed. New York: Basic Books, 2017.

Marsh, Frank H., and Janet Katz, eds. *Biology, Crime and Ethics: A Study of Biological Explanations for Criminal Behavior.* Cincinnati, OH: Anderson, 1984.

Mason, B. J. "New Threat to Blacks: Brain Surgery to Control Behavior—Controversial Operations Are Coming Back as Violence Curbs." *Ebony,* February 1973.

McCrory, Eamon, Joseph R. Ogle, Mattia Indi Gerin, and Essi Viding. "Neurocognitive Adaptation and Mental Health Vulnerability following Maltreatment: The Role of Social Functioning." *Child Maltreatment* 24, no. 4 (2019): 435–51.

M'charek, Amade. "Silent Witness, Articulate Collective: DNA Evidence and the Inference of Visible Traits." *Bioethics* 22, no. 9 (2008): 519–28.

M'charek, Amade, Katharina Schramm, and David Skinner. "Technologies of Belonging: The Absent Presence of Race in Europe." *Science, Technology, & Human Values* 39, no. 4 (2014): 459–67.

Mednick, Sarnoff A., William F. Gabrielli, and Barry Hutchings. "Genetic Influences in Criminal Convictions: Evidence from an Adoption Cohort." *Science* 224, no. 4651 (1984): 891–94.

Mednick, Sarnoff A., and Jan Volavka. "Biology and Crime." *Crime and Justice* 2 (1980): 85–158.

Merriman, Tony, and Vicky Cameron. "Risk-Taking: Behind the Warrior Gene Story." *New Zealand Medical Journal* 120, no. 1250 (2007): 1–4.

Messerschmidt, James W. *Crime as Structured Action: Doing Masculinities, Race, Class, Sexuality, and Crime.* Lanham, MD: Rowman & Littlefield, 2013.

―――. *Masculinities and Crime: Critique and Reconceptualization of Theory.* Lanham, MD: Rowman & Littlefield, 1993.

Metzl, Jonathan. *The Protest Psychosis: How Schizophrenia Became a Black Disease.* 6th ed.. Boston: Beacon Press, 2011.

Meyer-Lindenberg, Andreas. "From Maps to Mechanisms through Neuroimaging of Schizophrenia." *Nature* 468, no. 7321 (2010): 194–202.

Meyer-Lindenberg, Andreas, Joshua W. Buckholtz, Bhaskar Kolachana, Ahmad R. Hariri, Lukas Pezawas, Giuseppe Blasi, Ashley Wabnitz et al. "Neural Mechanisms of Genetic Risk for Impulsivity and Violence in Humans." *Proceedings of the National Academy of Sciences* 103, no. 16 (2006): 6269–74.

Mills, C. Wright. *The Sociological Imagination.* New York: Oxford University Press, 2000.

Moffitt, T. E. "Adolescence-Limited and Life-Course-Persistent Antisocial Behavior: A Developmental Taxonomy." *Psychological Review* 100, no. 4 (1993): 674–701.

Moran, Richard. "Biomedical Research and the Politics of Crime Control: A Historical Perspective." *Contemporary Crises* 2, no. 3 (1978): 335–57.

―――. "Medicine and Crime: The Search for the Born Criminal and the Medical Control of Criminality." In *Deviance and Medicalization: From Badness to Sickness*, edited by Peter Conrad and Joseph W. Schneider, 215–40. Philadelphia: Temple University Press, 1992.

Morell, V. "Evidence Found for a Possible 'Aggression Gene.'" *Science* 260, no. 5115 (1993): 1722–23.

Morning, Ann. *The Nature of Race: How Scientists Think and Teach about Human Difference.* Berkeley: University of California Press, 2011.

Muhammad, Khalil Gibran. *The Condemnation of Blackness: Race, Crime, and the Making of Modern Urban America.* 1st ed. Cambridge, MA: Harvard University Press, 2010.

Murphy, Erin E. "Familial DNA Searches: The Opposing Viewpoint." *Criminal Justice* 27, no. 1 (2012): 19–25.

Nadelhoffer, Thomas, and Walter Sinnott-Armstrong. "Neurolaw and Neuroprediction: Potential Promises and Perils." *Philosophy Compass* 7, no. 9 (2012): 631–42.

National Collaborating Centre for Mental Health (UK). *Antisocial Personality Disorder.* London: British Psychological Society, 2010.

National Commission for the Protection of Human Subjects of Biomedical and Behavioral Research. "Psychosurgery: Report and Recommendations." Bethesda, MD: U.S. Department of Health Education and Welfare (DHEW), 1977. https://videocast.nih.gov/pdf/ohrp_psychosurgery.pdf.

National Institutes of Health. "Genetics Home Reference: Gene Therapy." Lister Hill National Center for Biomedical Communications, October 1, 2019. U.S. National Library of Medicine. https://ghr.nlm.nih.gov/.

Nelkin, Dorothy, and M. Susan Lindee. *The DNA Mystique: The Gene as a Cultural Icon*. Ann Arbor: University of Michigan Press, 2010.

Nelkin, Dorothy, and Judith Swazey. "Science and Social Control." In *Violence and the Politics of Research*, edited by Willard Gaylin, Ruth Macklin, and Tabitha M. Powledge, 143–62. Hastings Center Series in Ethics. New York: Springer, 1981.

Nelson, Alondra. *Body and Soul: The Black Panther Party and the Fight against Medical Discrimination*. Minneapolis: University of Minnesota Press, 2012.

———. *The Social Life of DNA: Race, Reparations, and Reconciliation after the Genome*. 1st ed. Boston: Beacon Press, 2016.

2Nelson, Randy J. *Biology of Aggression*. Oxford, UK: Oxford University Press, 2006.

New York Times. "Extra Chromosome Brings an Acquittal on Murder Charge." October 10, 1968.

Niehoff, Debra. *The Biology of Violence: How Understanding the Brain, Behavior, and Encironment Can Break the Cycle of Violence*. 1st ed. New York: Free Press, 1999.

Novas, Carlos, and Nikolas Rose. "Genetic Risk and the Birth of the Somatic Individual." *Economy and Society* 29, no. 4 (2000): 485–513.

Nuechterlein, K. H., R. Parasuraman, and Q. Jiang. "Visual Sustained Attention: Image Degradation Produces Rapid Sensitivity Decrement over Time." *Science* 220, no. 4594 (1983): 327–29.

Obama, Barack. "Remarks by the President on the BRAIN Initiative and American Innovation." Presidential speech presented at the BRAIN Initiative, The White House, April 2, 2013. https://obamawhitehouse.archives.gov/the-press-office/2013/04/02/remarks-president-brain-initiative-and-american-innovation.

Obasogie, Osagie. *Blinded by Sight: Seeing Race through the Eyes of the Blind*. Stanford, CA: Stanford Law Books, 2013.

Ogloff, James R. P. "Psychopathy/Antisocial Personality Disorder Conundrum." *Australian and New Zealand Journal of Psychiatry* 40, no. 6–7 (2006): 519–28.

Omi, Michael, and Howard Winant. *Racial Formation in the United States*. 2nd ed. New York: Routledge, 1994.

Ossorio, Pilar, and Troy Duster. "Race and Genetics: Controversies in Biomedical, Behavioral, and Forensic Sciences." *American Psychologist* 60, no. 1 (2005): 115–28.

Pager, Devah. "The Mark of a Criminal Record." *American Journal of Sociology* 108, no. 5 (2003): 937–75.

Panofsky, Aaron. "Field Analysis and Interdisciplinary Science: Scientific Capital Exchange in Behavior Genetics." *Minerva* 49, no. 3 (2011):295–316

Panofsky, Aaron. *Misbehaving Science: Controversy and the Development of Behavior Genetics.* Chicago: University of Chicago Press, 2014.

People v. Tanner, 13 Cal. App. 3d 596 (Court of Appeals of California, Second District, Division Three, 1970).

Petteway, Ryan, Mahasin Mujahid, and Amani Allen. "Understanding Embodiment in Place-Health Research: Approaches, Limitations, and Opportunities." *Journal of Urban Health: Bulletin of the New York Academy of Medicine* 96, no. 2 (2019): 289–99.

Phelan, Jo C., and Bruce G. Link. "Is Racism a Fundamental Cause of Inequalities in Health?" *Annual Review of Sociology* 41, no. 1 (2015): 311–30.

Philipps, Axel, and Leonie Weißenborn. "Unconventional Ideas Conventionally Arranged: A Study of Grant Proposals for Exceptional Research." *Social Studies of Science* 49, no. 6 (2019): 884–97.

Pickersgill, M. D. "NICE Guidelines, Clinical Practice and Antisocial Personality Disorder: The Ethical Implications of Ontological Uncertainty." *Journal of Medical Ethics* 35, no. 11 (2009): 668–71.

Pickersgill, Martyn. "Between Soma and Society: Neuroscience and the Ontology of Psychopathy." *BioSocieties* 4, no. 1 (2009): 45–60.

———. "The Co-Production of Science, Ethics, and Emotion." *Science, Technology, & Human Values* 37, no. 6 (2012): 579–603.

———. "The Endurance of Uncertainty: Antisociality and Ontological Anarchy in British Psychiatry, 1950–2010." *Science in Context* 27, no. 1 (2014): 143–75.

———. "Ordering Disorder: Knowledge Production and Uncertainty in Neuroscience Research." *Science as Culture* 20, no. 1 (2011): 71–87.

———. "The Social Life of the Brain: Neuroscience in Society." *Current Sociology* 61, no. 3 (2013): 322–40.

———. "Standardising Antisocial Personality Disorder: The Social Shaping of a Psychiatric Technology." *Sociology of Health & Illness* 34, no. 4 (2012): 544–59.

Pietrini, Pietro, Mario Guazzelli, Gianpaolo Basso, Karen Jaffe, and Jordan Grafman. "Neural Correlates of Imaginal Aggressive Behavior Assessed by Positron Emission Tomography in Healthy Subjects." *American Journal of Psychiatry* 157, no. 11 (November 1, 2000): 1772–81.

Pinderhughes, Howard. *"Changing Landscapes of Violence through Social and Physical Interventions"* In *Community Violence as a Population Health Issue:*

Proceedings of a Workshop, edited by National Academies of Sciences, Engineering, and Medicine, 17-30. Washington, DC: National Academies Press, 2017.

———. *Race in the Hood: Conflict and Violence among Urban Youth*. 1st ed. Minneapolis: University of Minnesota Press, 1997.

Pinderhughes, Howard, Rachel Davis, and Myesha Williams. "Adverse Community Experiences and Resilience: A Framework for Addressing and Preventing Community Trauma." Oakland, CA: Prevention Institute, 2016.

Pitts-Taylor, Victoria. *The Brain's Body: Neuroscience and Corporeal Politics*. Durham, NC: Duke University Press, 2016.

———. "Neurobiologically Poor? Brain Phenotypes, Inequality, and Biosocial Determinism." *Science, Technology, & Human Values* 44, no. 4 (2019): 660–85.

Platt, Tony, and Paul Takagi. "Biosocial Criminology: A Critique." *Crime and Social Justice*, no. 11 (1979): 5–13.

Poldrack, Russell A. "Can Cognitive Processes Be Inferred from Neuroimaging Data?" *Trends in Cognitive Sciences* 10, no. 2 (February 2006): 59–63.

———. *The New Mind Readers: What Neuroimaging Can and Cannot Reveal about Our Thoughts*. Princeton, NJ: Princeton University Press, 2018.

Poldrack, Russell A., John Monahan, Peter B. Imrey, Valerie Reyna, Marcus E. Raichle, David Faigman, and Joshua W. Buckholtz. "Predicting Violent Behavior: What Can Neuroscience Add?" *Trends in Cognitive Sciences* 22, no. 2 (2018): 111–23.

Pollack, Seymour L. "Role of Brain Disease in Riots and Urban Violence." *Journal of the American Medical Association (JAMA)* 202, no. 7 (1967): 663.

Porter, Theodore M. *Trust in Numbers: The Pursuit of Objectivity in Science and Public Life*. Princeton, NJ: Princeton University Press, 1996.

Prainsack, Barbara, and Martin Kitzberger. "DNA behind Bars: Other Ways of Knowing Forensic DNA Technologies." *Social Studies of Science* 39, no. 1 (2009): 51–79.

Pretus, Clara, Nafees Hamid, Hammad Sheikh, Jeremy Ginges, Adolf Tobeña, Richard Davis, Oscar Vilarroya, and Scott Atran. "Neural and Behavioral Correlates of Sacred Values and Vulnerability to Violent Extremism." *Frontiers in Psychology* 9 (2018): 1–12.

Rafter, Nicole Hahn. *The Criminal Brain: Understanding Biological Theories of Crime*. New York: NYU Press, 2008.

———. "H. J. Eysenck in Fagin's Kitchen: The Return to Biological Theory in 20th-Century Criminology." *History of the Human Sciences* 19, no. 4 (2006): 37–56.

Raichle, Marcus E. "A Brief History of Human Brain Mapping." *Trends in Neurosciences* 32, no. 2 (2009): 118–26.

Raine, Adrian. *The Anatomy of Violence: The Biological Roots of Crime.* 1st ed. New York: Pantheon, 2013.

———. "Biosocial Studies of Antisocial and Violent Behavior in Children and Adults: A Review." *Journal of Abnormal Child Psychology* 30, no. 4 (2002): 311–26.

———. "From Genes to Brain to Antisocial Behavior." *Current Directions in Psychological Science* 17, no. 5 (2008): 323–28.

———. *The Psychopathology of Crime: Criminal Behavior as a Clinical Disorder.* 1st ed. San Diego: Academic Press, 1993.

Raine, Adrian, Patricia Brennan, David Farrington, and Sarnoff A. Mednick, "Biosocial Bases of Violence: Conceptual and Theoretical Issues." In *Biosocial Bases of Violence*, edited by Adrian Raine, Patricia Brennan, David Farrington, and Sarnoff A. Mednick, 1–20. New York: Springer, 1997.

Raine, Adrian, Monte Buchsbaum, and Lori Lacasse. "Brain Abnormalities in Murderers Indicated by Positron Emission Tomography." *Biological Psychiatry* 42, no. 6 (1997): 495–508.

Raine, Adrian, Monte S. Buchsbaum, Jill Stanley, Steven Lottenberg, Leonard Abel, and Jacqueline Stoddard. "Selective Reductions in Prefrontal Glucose Metabolism in Murderers." *Biological Psychiatry* 36, no. 6 (1994): 365–73.

Raine, Adrian, Todd Lencz, Susan Bihrle, Lori LaCasse, and Patrick Colletti. "Reduced Prefrontal Gray Matter Volume and Reduced Autonomic Activity in Antisocial Personality Disorder." *Archives of General Psychiatry* 57, no. 2 (2000): 119–27.

Raine, Adrian, Jianghong Liu, Peter H. Venables, Sarnoff A. Mednick, and C. Dalais. "Cohort Profile: The Mauritius Child Health Project." *International Journal of Epidemiology* 39, no. 6 (2010): 1441–51.

Raine, Adrian, J. Reid Meloy, Susan Bihrle, Jackie Stoddard, Lori LaCasse, and Monte S. Buchsbaum. "Reduced Prefrontal and Increased Subcortical Brain Functioning Assessed Using Positron Emission Tomography in Predatory and Affective Murderers." *Behavioral Sciences & the Law* 16, no. 3 (1998): 319–32.

Raine, Adrian, Jackie Stoddard, Susan Bihrle, and Monte Buchsbaum. "Prefrontal Glucose Deficits in Murderers Lacking Psychosocial Deprivation." *Neuropsychiatry, Neuropsychology, and Behavioral Neurology* 11, no. 1 (1998): 1–7.

Raine, Adrian, Peter H. Venables, Cyril Dalais, Kjetil Mellingen, Chandra Reynolds, and Sarnoff A. Mednick. "Early Educational and Health Enrichment at Age 3–5 Years Is Associated with Increased Autonomic and Central Nervous System Arousal and Orienting at Age 11 Years: Evidence from the Mauritius Child Health Project." *Psychophysiology* 38 (2001): 254–66.

Rajan, Kaushik Sunder. *Biocapital: The Constitution of Postgenomic Life*. Durham, NC: Duke University Press, 2006.

Ray, Victor, and Danielle Purifoy. "The Colorblind Organization." In *Race, Organizations, and the Organizing Process, edited by M. Wooten*, 131–50. Bingley, UK: Emerald Publishing, 2019.

Reardon, Jennifer. "The Democratic, Anti-Racist Genome? Technoscience at the Limits of Liberalism." *Science as Culture* 21, no. 1 (2012): 25–47.

———. *Race to the Finish: Identity and Governance in an Age of Genomics*. Princeton, NJ: Princeton University Press, 2005.

Remmel, Rheanna J., Andrea L. Glenn, and Jennifer Cox. "Biological Evidence regarding Psychopathy Does Not Affect Mock Jury Sentencing." *Journal of Personality Disorders* 33, no. 2 (2019): 164–84.

Rensberger, Boyce. "Science and Sensitivity." *Washington Post*, March 1, 1992. https://www.washingtonpost.com/archive/opinions/1992/03/01/science-and-sensitivity/285e7541-3b66-48c4-9cc9-55fb37d013f9/.

Riccio, Cynthia A, Cecil R Reynolds, Patricia Lowe, and Jennifer J. Moore. "The Continuous Performance Test: A Window on the Neural Substrates for Attention?" *Archives of Clinical Neuropsychology* 17, no. 3 (2002): 235–72.

Richardson, Sarah S. *Sex Itself: The Search for Male and Female in the Human Genome*. Chicago: University of Chicago Press, 2013.

Rijcke, Sarah de, and Anne Beaulieu. "Networked Neuroscience: Brain Scans and Visual Knowing at the Intersection of Atlases and Databases." In *Representation in Scientific Practice Revisited*, edited by Catelijne Coopmans, Janet Vertesi, Michael E. Lynch, and Steve Woolgar, 131–52. Cambridge, MA: MIT Press, 2014.

Rios, Victor M. *Punished: Policing the Lives of Black and Latino Boys*. New York: NYU Press, 2011.

Roberts, Dorothy E. *Fatal Invention: How Science, Politics, and Big Business Re-Create e in the Twenty-First Century*. New York: New Press, 2011.

———. *Killing the Black Body: Race, Reproduction, and the Meaning of Liberty*. New York: Vintage Books, 1999.

———. "Law, Race, and Biotechnology: Toward a Biopolitical and Transdisciplinary Paradigm." *Annual Review of Law and Social Science* 9, no. 1 (2013): 149–66.

Roberts, Dorothy E., and Oliver Rollins. "Why Sociology Matters to Race and Biosocial Science." *Annual Review of Sociology* 46, no. 1 (2020): 195–214.

Rollins, Oliver E. "Risky Bodies: Race and the Science of Crime and Violence." In *Living Racism: Through the Barrel of the Book*, edited by Theresa Rajack-Talley and Derrick R. Brooms, 97–119. Lanham, MD: Lexington Books, 2018.

Rose, Nikolas. *The Politics of Life Itself: Biomedicine, Power, and Subjectivity in the Twenty-First Century*. Princeton, NJ: Princeton University Press, 2007.

———. "'Screen and Intervene': Governing Risky Brains." *History of the Human Sciences* 23, no. 1 (2010): 79–105.

Rose, Nikolas, and Joelle M. Abi-Rached. *Neuro: The New Brain Sciences and the Management of the Mind*. Princeton, NJ: Princeton University Press, 2013.

Roskies, Adina L. "Neuroimaging and Inferential Distance." *Neuroethics* 1, no. 1 (2008): 19–30.

Rosvold, Enger H., Allan F. Mirsky, Irwin Sarason, Edwin D. Bransome Jr., and Lloyd H. Beck. "A Continuous Performance Test of Brain Damage." *Journal of Consulting Psychology* 20, no. 5 (1956): 343–50.

Roth, Wendy D., and Biorn Ivemark. "Genetic Options: The Impact of Genetic Ancestry Testing on Consumers' Racial and Ethnic Identities." *American Journal of Sociology* 124, no. 1 (2018): 150–84.

Royce, Kenneth. *The XYY Man*. London: Hodder & Stoughton, 1970.

Rubin, Beatrix P. "Therapeutic Promise in the Discourse of Human Embryonic Stem Cell Research." *Science as Culture* 17, no. 1 (2008): 13–27.

Sampson, Robert J., and John H. Laub. "A Life-Course View of the Development of Crime." *The ANNALS of the American Academy of Political and Social Science* 602, no. 1 (2005): 12–45.

Scheinost, Dustin, Stephanie Noble, Corey Horien, Abigail S. Greene, Evelyn MR. Lake, Mehraveh Salehi, Siyuan Gao et al. "Ten Simple Rules for Predictive Modeling of Individual Differences in Neuroimaging." *NeuroImage* 193 (2019): 35–45.

Scurich, Nicholas, and Adam Shniderman. "The Selective Allure of Neuroscientific Explanations." *PLoS ONE* 9, no. 9 (2014).

Selk, Avi. "The Ingenious and 'Dystopian' DNA Technique Police Used to Hunt the 'Golden State Killer' Suspect." *Washington Post*, April 28, 2018, True Crime section. https://www.washingtonpost.com/news/true-crime/wp/2018/04/27/golden-state-killer-dna-website-gedmatch-was-used-to-identify-joseph-deangelo-as-suspect-police-say/.

Shapin, Steven, and Simon Schaffer. *Leviathan and the Air-Pump: Hobbes, Boyle, and the Experimental Life*. Reprint ed. Princeton, NJ: Princeton University Press, 2011.

Shen, Francis X. "The Overlooked History of Neurolaw Symposium: Criminal Behavior and the Brain: When Law and Neuroscience Collide." *Fordham Law Review*, no. 2 (2016): 667–96.

Shih, J. C., and K. Chen. "MAO-A and -B Gene Knock-out Mice Exhibit Distinctly Different Behavior." *Neurobiology (Budapest, Hungary)* 7, no. 2 (1999): 235–46.

Shim, Janet K. "Bio-Power and Racial, Class, and Gender Formation in Biomedical Knowledge Production." In *Research in the Sociology of Health*, edited by J. J. Kronenfeld, 173–95. Stamford, CT: JAI Press, 2000.

———. *Heart-Sick: The Politics of Risk, Inequality, and Heart Disease*. New York: NYU Press, 2014.

Shim, Janet K., Sonia Rab Alam, and Bradley E. Aouizerat. "Knowing Something versus Feeling Different: The Effects and Non-Effects of Genetic Ancestry on Racial Identity." *New Genetics and Society* 37, no. 1 (2018): 44–66.

Siever, Larry J. "Neurobiology of Aggression and Violence." *American Journal of Psychiatry* 165, no. 4 (2008): 429–42.

Silva, Kumarini. *Brown Threat: Identification in the Security State*. Minneapolis: University of Minnesota Press, 2016.

Simon, Jonathan. "Positively Punitive: How the Inventor of Scientific Criminology Who Died at the Beginning of the Twentieth Century Continues to Haunt American Crime Control at the Beginning of the Twenty-First." *Texas Law Review* 84 (2006): 2135–72.

Star, Susan L. *Regions of the Mind: Brain Research and the Quest for Scientific Certainty*. Stanford, CA: Stanford University Press, 1989.

Star, Susan L, and Anselm Strauss. "Layers of Silence, Arenas of Voice: The Ecology of Visible and Invisible Work." *Computer Supported Cooperative Work (CSCW)* 8, no. 1 (1999): 9–30.

Stepan, Nancy. *The Idea of Race in Science: Great Britain, 1800–1960*. 1st U.S. ed. Hamden, CT: Archon, 1982.

Sterzer, Philipp, Christina Stadler, Annette Krebs, Andreas Kleinschmidt, and Fritz Poustka. "Abnormal Neural Responses to Emotional Visual Stimuli in Adolescents with Conduct Disorder." *Biological Psychiatry* 57, no. 1 (2005): 7–15.

Stochholm, Kirstine, Anders Bojesen, Anne Skakkebæk Jensen, Svend Juul, and Claus Højbjerg Gravholt. "Criminality in Men with Klinefelter's Syndrome and XYY Syndrome: A Cohort Study." *BMJ Open* 2, no. 1 (2012): e000650.

Stock, Robert W. "The XYY and the Criminal." *New York Times,* October 20, 1968.

Strauss, Anselm L. *Continual Permutations of Action*. New Brunswick, NJ: AldineTransaction, 2008.

Taylor Jr., Stuart. "Cat Scans Said to Show Shrunken Hinckley Brain." *New York Times*, June 2, 1982, section D.

———. "Hinckley's Brain Is Termed Normal." *New York Times,* June 4, 1982, section A.

————. "Judge Rebukes Hinckley Witness over Cat Scan." *New York Times*, May 20, 1982, section B.

Thompson, Charis. *Making Parents: The Ontological Choreography of Reproductive Technologies*. Cambridge, MA: MIT Press, 2005.

Timmermans, Stefan. "Matching Genotype and Phenotype: A Pragmatist Semiotic Analysis of Clinical Exome Sequencing." *American Journal of Sociology* 123, no. 1 (2017): 136–77.

Timmermans, Stefan, and Steven Epstein. "A World of Standards but Not a Standard World: Toward a Sociology of Standards and Standardization." *Annual Review of Sociology* 36, no. 1 (2010): 69–89.

Tolwinski, Kasia. "Fraught Claims at the Intersection of Biology and Sociality: Managing Controversy in the Neuroscience of Poverty and Adversity." *Social Studies of Science* 49, no. 2 (2019): 141–61.

Tomlinson, Rachel C., S. Alexandra Burt, Rebecca Waller, John Jonides, Alison L. Miller, Ashley N. Gearhardt, Scott J. Peltier, Kelly L. Klump, Julie C. Lumeng, and Luke W. Hyde. "Neighborhood Poverty Predicts Altered Neural and Behavioral Response Inhibition." *NeuroImage* 209 (2020): 1–9.

Umhau, John C., Karysse Trandem, Mohsin Shah, and David T. George. "The Physician's Unique Role in Preventing Violence: A Neglected Opportunity?" *BMC Medicine* 10 (2012): 146.

Uttal, William R. *The New Phrenology: The Limits of Localizing Cognitive Processes in the Brain*. Cambridge, MA: MIT Press, 2001.

Valenstein, Elliot S. *The Psychosurgery Debate: Scientific, Legal, and Ethical Perspectives*. San Francisco: W. H. Freeman, 1980.

Vassos, E., D. A. Collier, and S. Fazel. "Systematic Meta-Analyses and Field Synopsis of Genetic Association Studies of Violence and Aggression." *Molecular Psychiatry* 19, no. 4 (2014): 471–77.

Vidal, Fernando. "Brainhood, Anthropological Figure of Modernity." *History of the Human Sciences* 22, no. 1 (2009): 5–36.

————. "What Makes Neuroethics Possible?" *History of the Human Sciences* 32, no. 2 (2018): 32–58.

Viding, Essi, and Eamon McCrory. "Genetic Biomarker Research of Callous-Unemotional Traits in Children: Implications for the Law and Policymaking." In *Bioprediction, Biomarkers, and Bad Behavior: Scientific, Legal, and Ethical Challenges*, edited by Ilina Singh, Walter Sinnott-Armstrong, and Julian Savulecu, 153–72. New York: Oxford University Press, 2014.

————. "Why Should We Care about Measuring Callous-Unemotional Traits in Children?" *British Journal of Psychiatry: The Journal of Mental Science* 200, no. 3 (2012): 177–78.

Volavka, Jan. *Neurobiology of Violence.* 2nd ed. Washington, DC: American Psychiatric Publishing, 2002.

Volkow, Nora D., George F. Koob, and A. Thomas McLellan. "Neurobiologic Advances from the Brain Disease Model of Addiction." *New England Journal of Medicine* 374, no. 4 (2016): 363–71.

Volkow, Nora D., and Laurence Tancredi. "Neural Substrates of Violent Behaviour: A Preliminary Study with Positron Emission Tomography." *British Journal of Psychiatry* 151, no. 5 (1987): 668–73.

Wacquant, Loïc. "From Slavery to Mass Incarceration: Rethinking the 'Race Question' in the US." *New Left Review* 13 (2002): 41–60.

———. *Punishing the Poor: The Neoliberal Government of Social Insecurity.* Durham, NC: Duke University Press, 2009.

Wade, Peter. *Race and Ethnicity in Latin America.* 2nd ed. New York: Pluto Press, 2010.

Wailoo, Keith, Alondra Nelson, and Catherine Lee, eds. *Genetics and the Unsettled Past: The Collision of DNA, Race, and History.* New Brunswick, NJ: Rutgers University Press, 2012.

Walby, Kevin, and Nicolas Carrier. "The Rise of Biocriminology: Capturing Observable Bodily Economies of 'Criminal Man.'" *Criminology & Criminal Justice* 10, no. 3 (2010): 261–85.

Walker, Renee E., Christopher R. Keane, and Jessica G. Burke. "Disparities and Access to Healthy Food in the United States: A Review of Food Deserts Literature." *Health & Place* 16, no. 5 (2010): 876–84.

Walsh, Charlotte. "Youth Justice and Neuroscience: A Dual-Use Dilemma." *British Journal of Criminology* 51, no. 1 (2011): 21–39.

Ward, Geoff. "The Slow Violence of State Organized Race Crime." *Theoretical Criminology* 19, no. 3 (2015): 299–314.

Wasserman, David, and Robert Wachbroit, eds. *Genetics and Criminal Behavior.* Cambridge, UK: Cambridge University Press, 2001.

Weheliye, Alexander G. *Habeas Viscus: Racializing Assemblages, Biopolitics, and Black Feminist Theories of the Human.* Durham, NC: Duke University Press, 2014.

Weinberg, Alvin. "Science and Trans-Science." *Minerva* 10, no. 2 (1974): 209–22.

Weisberg, Deena Skolnick, Frank C. Keil, Joshua Goodstein, Elizabeth Rawson, and Jeremy R. Gray. "The Seductive Allure of Neuroscience Explanations." *Journal of Cognitive Neuroscience* 20, no. 3 (2008): 470–77.

Weisberg, Deena Skolnick, Jordan C. V. Taylor, and Emily J. Hopkins. "Deconstructing the Seductive Allure of Neuroscience Explanations." *Judgment and Decision Making; Tallahassee* 10, no. 5 (2015): 429–41.

Wetzell, Richard F. "Criminology in Weimar and Nazi Germany." In *Criminals and Their Scientists: The History of Criminology in International Perspective*, edited by Peter Becker and Richard F. Wetzell. 1st ed. New York: Cambridge University Press, 2006.

Whitmarsh, Ian, and David S. Jones. *What's the Use of Race?: Modern Governance and the Biology of Difference*. Cambridge, MA: MIT Press, 2010.

Williams, David R., Jourdyn A. Lawrence, and Brigette A. Davis. "Racism and Health: Evidence and Needed Research." *Annual Review of Public Health* 40, no. 1 (2019): 105–25.

Witkin, Herman A., Sarnoff A. Mednick, Fini Schulsinger, Eskild Bakkestrøm, Karl O. Christiansen, Donald R. Goodenough, Kurt Hirschhorn et al. "Criminality in XYY and XXY Men." *Science* 193, no. 4253 (1976): 547–55.

Young, Rebecca M., and Evan Balaban. "Aggression, Biology, and Context." In *Neurobiology of Aggression: Understanding and Preventing Violence*, edited by Mark P. Mattson, 191–211. Contemporary Neuroscience. Totowa, NJ: Humana Press, 2003.

Yudell, Michael. *Race Unmasked: Biology and Race in the Twentieth Century*. New York: Columbia University Press, 2014.

Zaalberg, Ap, Henk Nijman, Erik Bulten, Luwe Stroosma, and Cees van der Staak. "Effects of Nutritional Supplements on Aggression, Rule-Breaking, and Psychopathology among Young Adult Prisoners." *Aggressive Behavior* 36, no. 2 (2010): 117–26.

Zuberi, Tukufu. *Thicker Than Blood: How Racial Statistics Lie*. Minneapolis: University of Minnesota Press, 2001.

Zuberi, Tukufu, and Eduardo Bonilla-Silva, eds. *White Logic, White Methods: Racism and Methodology*. Lanham, MD: Rowman & Littlefield, 2008.

Index

of, 21, 124, 136–43, 155–56; production and legitimation of, 9–12, 49; qualification of measures in, 41–44; race in relation to, ix–x, 20–21, 108–22; and racism, 119–20; research program ("the program") on, 6–15, 17–21, 149–50; risk for violence as topic of, 15; role of "the social" in, 9–10, 12–14, 17, 19, 20, 22, 96, 118–19, 148–51, 155–58; subjects of study for, 32–36, 69–70, 168n40; therapeutic promise of, 21, 25, 124–30, 141, 145, 148, 151, 153; uncertainty, complexity, and controversy in, 7, 9–14, 18–19, 21, 27–32, 44, 58–59, 64, 68, 98–99, 147–48; utility of, xii, 29–30, 155. *See also* risk/vulnerability, for violence

New York Times (newspaper), 47, 80

Niehoff, Deborah, 12, 14

NIH. *See* U.S. National Institutes of Health

normality: criteria for determination of, 69–72; environmental/social factors and, 95–96; violent/antisocial proclivities contrasted with, 11, 95–96; violent brain model in relation to, 17, 19, 69–73

Novas, Carlos, 133–34

nutrition, 130, 184n34

Obama, Barack, 6

objectivity: in evaluation of risk potential of individuals, 14, 15; medicalization and, 24; quantification linked to, 40–41; in risk calculations, 15; visual representation linked to, 53, 63–64, 139

oppositional defiant disorder (ODD), 37

Panofsky, Aaron, 10, 98, 167n37

Pardini, Dustin, 27–28

parenting, 133–36, 143

Parker, Barrington, 46–47

Pavlov, Ivan, 24

PCL-R. *See* Psychopathy Checklist

People v. Tanner, 81

personality, linked to crime, 23–24

personhood. *See* subjectivity/personhood

PET. *See* positron emission tomography (PET)

Pickersgill, Martyn, 32, 39

Pitts-Taylor, Victoria, 135

Poldrack, Russell, 57

Pollack, Seymour, 103

Porter, Theodore, 40–41

positron emission tomography (PET), 56, 57, 59, 60, 108. *See also* neuroimaging

Poussaint, Alvin, 103–4

poverty, 103, 120, 135

prefrontal cortex, 43, 58, 120, 137, 157

prison populations: embrace of violent brain model by, 129; psychopathology in, 33; as subjects of study, 32–36, 168n40

progress, x–xii, 17–18, 50

promissory value, 126, 148

psychopathy, 37, 39–42, 63

Psychopathy Checklist (PCL-R), 39–41

psychosurgery, 102–5, 123

race: absent presence of, 20–21, 108–10, 112, 163n54; biological approaches to, viii, x, 20; biology

Printed in the USA
CPSIA information can be obtained
at www.ICGtesting.com
JSHW021617200124
55658JS00021B/216

9 781503 627895